ADAPTATION TO LOSS
through
Short-Term
Group
Psychotherapy

ADAPTATION TO LOSS

through Short-Term Group Psychotherapy

WILLIAM E. PIPER
MARY MCCALLUM
HASSAN F. A. AZIM

University of Alberta and
University of Alberta Hospitals

THE GUILFORD PRESS
New York   London

© 1992 The Guilford Press
A Division of Guilford Publications, Inc.
72 Spring Street, New York 10012

Printed in the United States of America

This book is printed on acid-free paper.

Last digit is print number: 9 8 7 6 5 4 3 2 1

Library of Congress Cataloging-in-Publication Data

Piper, William E.
  Adaptation to loss through short-term group psychotherapy /
William E. Piper, Mary McCallum, Hassan F. A. Azim.
     p.   cm.
  Includes bibliographical references and index.
  ISBN 0-89862-796-6
  1. Grief therapy. 2. Group psychotherapy. 3. Loss (Psychology)
I. McCallum, Mary, Ph.D. II. Azim, Hassan F. A. III. Title.
  [DNLM: 1. Grief. 2. Psychotherapy, Group—methods. BF 575.G7
P665a]
RC455.4.L67P56 1992
616.85′2—dc20
DNLM/DLC   92-1424
for Library of Congress   CIP

*To our patients and colleagues, who have provided inspiration
for this book.*

*To my wife, Martha, my daughters, Emily and Hannah,
and my mother, Margaret, who has experienced more
than her share of life's losses—W.E.P.*

*To my husband, Don, for his much appreciated support
and encouragement throughout the writing
of this book—M.M.*

*To my wife, Norma, and my three sons,
Ramsey, Omar, and Dean, for all
their support—H.F.A.A.*

Preface

This book is about a form of treatment for patients who, for a variety of reasons, have not adapted well to the loss of one or more persons. The treatment modality is time-limited, short-term group psychotherapy. The therapy groups are part of the Short-Term Group Therapy Program for Loss Patients, which operates within the Division of External Psychiatric Services, University of Alberta Hospitals, Edmonton, Alberta, Canada. Since 1986 over 25 loss groups have been conducted. Like other programs offered by the division, it was initiated in response to a pressing demand for services, in this case from patients who were experiencing difficulties associated with loss.

The treatment is defined as therapy rather than counseling, on both theoretical and technical grounds. Theoretically, its objectives include identifying internal conflicts that impede normal mourning processes and making internal changes that facilitate better adaptation to loss. Technically, clarification and interpretation are emphasized relative to support and direction, and immediate events in the group, such as the interaction among members, receive considerable attention. The general orientation of treatment is psychodynamic, with an emphasis on the group as a system. The participants of the groups are regarded as patients because most fulfill criteria for psychiatric diagnoses according to formal classification categories, and all are referred to, or request assistance at our outpatient psychiatry clinic. The losses are usually multiple and have been the result of death, separation, and/or divorce. They typically span the entire lives of the patients. The precipitating event has usually been a loss during the past year.

A unique feature of the short-term group program has been the inclusion of a controlled, clinical trial evaluation of the treatment. The study involved 16 of the therapy groups and 154 of the patients who were referred to the program. It utilized state-of-the-art procedures for conducting clinical trials. These included random allocation of patients to immediate or delayed therapy, verification of the treatment technique, experienced therapists, a large patient sample, a comprehensive battery of outcome measures, investigation of patient–treatment interactions, investigation of process–outcome relationships, and follow-up assessments. The results of the study revealed a strong treatment effect according to both statistical and clinical criteria. The project also identified a patient personality characteristic (psychological mindedness) that was significantly related to remaining and working in the groups.

In our opinion the findings of the project clearly enhance confidence in the efficacy of short-term psychotherapy groups. Of equal importance is that the project demonstrates that clinical and research tasks can be integrated in an active clinical setting to serve the interests of patients, clinicians, and researchers. For that reason the procedures associated with the project will be carefully elucidated along with the findings.

The introduction to the book describes how the Short-Term Group Therapy Program originated and considers some of its working assumptions about loss, persons experiencing loss, the role of psychotherapy, and clinical research. Chapter 1 reviews epidemiologic data concerning the magnitude of person losses and associated problems. It also considers conceptual issues, such as the distinction between normal and abnormal reactions to loss. In Chapter 2 some of the major psychoanalytic theories concerning pathologic grief are summarized. Chapter 3[1] considers various societal changes that have affected the resources available to people who suffer person losses. A simple conceptual framework for classifying stages and types of mourning is offered and used to review individual and group intervention methods.

Next, the Short-Term Loss Group Program and its primary components are addressed. Chapter 4[2] focuses on patient selection and preparation. With regard to selection, risk factors and indications of pathologic grief are reviewed. Two cases are used to illustrate characteristics that were found to be associated with success and failure in the loss groups. Next, several different approaches to preparation are described. Finally, exclusion criteria are presented. Chapter 5[3] addresses group composition and therapist technique as implemented in the Short-Term Loss Group Program. Homogeneity of group composition is emphasized. As to therapist technique, the concepts of interpretation and transference are discussed as precursors to describing the therapist's role in the loss groups. Consistent focus upon commonalities and productive use of limited time and the group (rather than individual) therapy situation are cited as cardinal features of the therapist's role.

The evolution of one group of the research project is followed in Chapter 6[4]. The concepts of theme and role are defined and used to chart the course of the group. The representativeness of many of the features of the group is emphasized. Chapter 7[5] reviews previous research that has evaluated the efficacy of group interventions for those who have experienced person losses. Recognition of certain limitations associated with previous research guided the methodology of the clinical trial research project, which is presented next in the book. Chapter 8[6] is devoted to a description of the project and presentation of its main outcome findings. Chapter 9[7] follows with a presentation of findings associated with the patient personality characteristic known as psychological mindedness and the patient performance characteristic known as psychodynamic work. The data concerning these two concepts provide insight into some of the mechanisms that may underlie dynamically oriented short-term group therapy. Finally, Chapter 10 addresses conclusions and future directions as well as limitations associated with the Short-Term Loss Group Program and the clinical trial research project.

Based upon what is covered, we believe that our book is relevant to the large community of mental health practitioners who provide services to psychiatric outpatients. That includes staff of public and private clinics as well as individual practitioners. Such professionals typically come from the disciplines of psychiatry, psychology, social work, occupational therapy, and nursing. These are the very disciplines represented in our clinic and hence the Short-Term Loss Group Program. The book is, of course, relevant to practitioners who are particularly interested in group forms of psychotherapy and/or problems associated with person loss. There is a strong emphasis on clinical research. We believe that this is particularly appropriate in view of the vocal demands of policy makers, third-party payers, and consumers for the validation of the efficacy of all therapeutic procedures. The research project that involved 16 of the groups clearly provides support for the conclusions reached about the clinical procedures. Moreover, we believe that the book describes an exciting collaborative process wherein clinicians and researchers succeeded in informing each other about their work, thus increasing each other's knowledge. Accordingly, we hope that the book might be useful to clinicians and researchers who are interested in the evaluation of treatment methods and therapeutic programs. The research project has been one of four similar recent studies in the Division of External Psychiatric Services of the University of Alberta Hospitals that have evaluated the effectiveness of ongoing programs.

The implementation of a clinical research project and a therapy program requires the collaboration of many people. To those directly involved with the project and program we wish to express our thanks and appreciation for their contribution. The therapists in the research project, in addition to M. M., were J. Fyfe Bahrey and William J. M. Nickerson. The research coordinator for the entire course of the project was Hillary L. Morin. She worked closely with several research assistants who included Jayne Carlielle, Ellen L. Perrault, Vuokko van der Veen, and L. Jill Zimmerman. Daniel S. K. Szeto served as our statistical consultant. In the clinic we are grateful for the support of the Service Chief of the Walk-in Clinic, Robert S. Lakoff. We also appreciate the support of the former chairman of the Department of Psychiatry, William G. Dewhurst, and the current chairman, Roger C. Bland. A number of therapists from the Walk-in Clinic participated in the weekly seminar that served as a seminal forum for the exchange of theoretical, clinical, and research ideas since the program's inception. They included Andrea L. Baggaley, Kristine M. Barone-Adesi, Sherryl L. Basarab, Sandra J. Dmytrash, Scott C. Duncan, Barbara N. Feist, Diane L. Holowachuk, Anthony S. Joyce, Linda L. McAuley, Roderick J. Misunis, Joan Newman, and Janis G. Thorkelssen. We also wish to thank Colleen S. Poon, who meticulously typed and prepared the manuscript.

The research project was supported by an operating grant (number 6609-142646) from the National Health Research and Development Program, Health and Welfare Canada; an operating grant (number 55-01502) from the Canadian Psychiatric Research Foundation; and an equipment grant (number 115-3) from the Special Services and Research Committee, University of Alberta Hospitals.

NOTES

1. Portions of Chapter 3 appear in the following publications: Lakoff, R. S., & Azim, H. F. A. (1991). Society's changing views on mourning: Some clinical implications. *Group Analysis*, 24, 355–362. Copyright by the Group-Analytic Society (London). Reprinted by permission. Piper, W. E., & McCallum, M. (1991). Group interventions for persons who have experienced loss: Description and evaluative research. *Group Analysis*, 24, 363–373. Copyright by the Group-Analytic Society. (London). Reprinted by permission.

2. Portions of Chapter 4 appear in McCallum, M., & Piper, W. E. (1988). Psychoanalytically oriented short-term groups for outpatients: Unsettled issues. *Group*, 12, 21–32. Copyright 1988 by the Eastern Group Psychotherapy Society. Reprinted by permission.

3. Portions of Chapter 5 appear in McCallum, M., & Piper, W. E. (1988). Psychoanalytically oriented short-term groups for outpatients: Unsettled issues. *Group, 12,* 21–32. Copyright 1988 by the Eastern Group Psychotherapy Society. Reprinted by permission.

4. Portions of Chapter 6 appear in the following publications: McCallum, M., Piper, W. E., Azim, H. F. A., & Lakoff, R. S. (1991). The Edmonton model of short-term group therapy for loss: An integration of theory, practice, and research. *Group Analysis, 24,* 375–388. Bahrey, J. F., McCallum, M., & Piper, W. E. (1991). Emergent themes and roles in short-term loss groups. *International Journal of Group Psychotherapy, 41,* 329–345. Copyright 1991 by the American Group Psychotherapy Association, Inc. Reprinted by permission.

5. Portions of Chapter 7 appear in Piper, W. E., & McCallum, M. (1991). Group interventions for persons who have experienced loss: Description and evaluative research. *Group Analysis, 24* 363–373. Copyright 1991 by the Group-Analytic Society (London). Reprinted by permission.

6. Portions of Chapter 8 appear in McCallum, M., & Piper, W. E. (1990). A controlled study of effectiveness and patient suitability for short-term group psychotherapy. *International Journal of Group Psychotherapy, 40,* 431–452. Copyright 1990 by the American Group Psychotherapy Association, Inc. Reprinted by permission.

7. Portions of Chapter 9 appear in McCallum, M., & Piper, W. E. (1990). The psychological mindedness assessment procedure. *Psychological Assessment: A Journal of Consulting and Clinical Psychology, 2,* 412–418. Copyright 1990 by the American Psychological Association, Inc. Reprinted by permission.

Contents

*ADAPTATION
TO LOSS*
*through
Short-Term
Group
Psychotherapy*

Introduction

In the fall of 1986, we initiated a treatment program in our clinic for psychiatric outpatients who were experiencing difficulties adapting to the loss of one or more persons. It was named the Short-Term Group Therapy Program for Loss Patients. The program is located within the Walk-in Clinic of the Division of External Psychiatric Services, University of Alberta Hospitals. The division is a large, multifaceted outpatient service for psychiatric patients that is located within an 800-bed university hospital. The Walk-in Clinic is a high-volume service that handles approximately 2,400 initial assessments each year. The clinical staff of the division is composed of professionals from the disciplines of psychiatry, psychology, social work, occupational therapy, and nursing. A variety of treatment alternatives including individual, couple, family, and group therapy; psychopharmacology; and partial hospitalization are provided.

The decision to create a special program for loss patients was influenced by several factors. As part of the ongoing service evaluations conducted in the division since its inception in 1973, a decision was made to review the program for short-term therapy groups. The groups were heterogeneous in patient composition and psychodynamically oriented. Our findings yielded several distinct impressions: (1) From the perspectives of the patients and therapists, the process and outcome of the groups were highly variable. Some progressed smoothly and were evaluated positively, whereas others floundered and led to questionable outcomes. Some suffered from significant attrition. (2) Issues associated with losses in the patients' lives and their consequences were frequently brought up in the groups. (3) The objectives of the groups were numerous and diverse. For the patient, they included symptom reduction, support, crisis

1

resolution, problem solving, psychological understanding of internal conflicts and patterns of interaction with others, and personality change. For the clinical staff, they also included student training, and both assessment and preparation for long-term group therapy. To the evaluation staff, it seemed that the groups were suffering from task overload, which had compromised the ability of several groups to provide effective treatment. In forming these impressions and making plans about future programs, we began to envision therapy groups that would have a more limited, but more realistic, set of objectives. That view was also influenced by developments in the field of short-term psychotherapy.

From the literature concerning short-term individual psychotherapy, we were aware of recommendations from a number of people to maintain a definite focus in therapy (Davanloo, 1978; Malan, 1976; Sifneos, 1979). This has usually been defined as a focal conflict, that is, a central repetitive conflict that has characterized important events, often entire periods, of a patient's life. It made good sense to us that a short-term form of therapy cannot deal thoroughly with all significant conflicts in a patient's life, but may be able to deal thoroughly with a focal conflict. We were also aware of forms of time-limited individual therapy that emphasize the limitations of life (Mann, 1973). The relevance of such limitations to persons suffering from loss was readily apparent. From the less extensive literature concerning short-term group therapy, we were aware of approaches that recommend homogeneous patient composition (Budman, Bennett, & Wisneski, 1981). The degree to which patient commonalities can facilitate cohesion and universality (a sense of shared experience) seemed to us to be of considerable potential value to short-term group approaches to therapy. Thus, issues concerning focality, time limitations, and patient homogeneity converged with our impressions of difficulties associated with the ongoing short-term therapy groups in our clinic.

What emerged from the process was a model for conducting time-limited, short-term therapy groups for loss patients. The groups were to focus upon issues related to loss, be conducted for a limited period of time (12 weeks), and be homogeneous with respect to several patient criteria. The more obvious criteria were to include loss itself and familiar associated feelings such as sadness and anger. The less obvious were to include problematic unresolved conflicts. In the spring of 1986, a pilot program for conducting such groups was started. This included establishment of a weekly seminar for a small number of interested clinicians and researchers, and a trial group led by two of them. Both the seminar and trial group went extremely well. Consequently, a more formalized program was presented to and accepted by the clinic staff and officially began in the fall of that year. From the beginning, the program also included plans and provided a structure for conducting formal evaluation of the groups. That feature had the effect of instilling a climate of inquiry and discovery in the program, which has persisted throughout. Applications for external funds to support a formal evaluation project were made and successfully obtained from two federal granting agencies (Health and Welfare Canada and the Canadian Psychiatric Research Foundation) for a 4-year period. The project, a controlled clinical trial, began in early 1987.

All treatment programs operate according to a set of working assumptions. Some are explicit, whereas others are implicit. They usually stem from multiple sources. Some assumptions are a product of affiliation with a particular theoretical and technical orientation. Others are a function of the practical demands of one's clinical setting, including the nature of the patients who seek assistance. Still others are determined by the value one attributes to clinical research and its relationship to clinical practice. Some working assumptions can be justified upon the basis of theoretical position, clinical practice, or research evidence, whereas others can be described as intuitive. Regardless of their source or the extent of their logical/empirical grounding, we believe that they exert a powerful influence on the structure and process of clinical programs.

In the case of the Short-Term Group Therapy Program for Loss Patients, several of the sources of its working assumptions have been evident. Its theoretical and technical orientation is psychodynamic and systemic. Thus, it encompasses both the traditional emphasis upon frequently unconscious and conflictual components (wishes, fears, defenses) at several levels (intrapsychic, interpersonal, intragroup) and the more recent emphasis upon object relationships. It also places emphasis upon the technique of interpretation. The program's location within a busy outpatient clinic meant that it had to be responsive to a large demand for service. At the same time, it was able to offer a specialized service because a variety of treatment options were available in the clinic. The leadership's commitment to the integration of clinical service and clinical research meant that research procedures were a routine part of activities of the division, including this program.

The following sections are intended to present a number of the working assumptions of the program. Some will receive considerable elaboration in the chapters that follow. We believe that an awareness of such assumptions at the beginning of this book will assist the reader in understanding and integrating the material presented in the various individual chapters.

ASSUMPTIONS ABOUT LOSS

Experiencing loss is an inevitable part of life. The losses of people, especially of those with whom we have established meaningful relationships, are among the most significant kinds of losses. Loss is a painful experience that includes symptomatic features. If those features were present in the absence of loss, they would usually indicate emotional disturbance. The distinction between normal and abnormal reactions to loss is ambiguous. Experts disagree. Nevertheless, extreme symptomatic manifestations, prolonged symptomatic manifestations, and the absence of symptoms altogether are commonly regarded as abnormal reactions. As one ages, the number of losses in one's life generally increases. Associated with each loss are permanent effects, some of which remain outside of conscious experience. Reactions to recent losses that seem out of proportion to the event are sometimes indicative of the cumulative effect of a number of losses. It is doubtful whether anyone fully resolves the loss of people, or is ever totally free of the effects of such losses.

ASSUMPTIONS ABOUT PERSONS
EXPERIENCING LOSS

People's reactions to loss are highly individual. Such reactions include defensive (adaptive as well as maladaptive) mechanisms and a spectrum of intensity and duration of symptomatic features. Responses to loss are also influenced by stable factors such as one's personality and the quality of object relations. An important determinant is how well a person has dealt with long-standing conflicts over such issues as trust, dependence, intimacy, and aggression. Responses to loss are also influenced by the specific nature of recent and past losses. A highly conflicted and ambivalent relationship with the lost person is prognostic of problematic reactions. People's needs following loss are also highly individual, although some need for catharsis and support appears to be universal. Traditionally, family, friends, and religious acquaintances have responded to such needs. Today there is reason to suspect that less support is being provided by such traditional resources, and that the growth of self-help and mutual-help organizations is perhaps due to an attempt to fill the resulting void. Most people suffering from loss do not request assistance from mental health clinics or mental health workers. Of those patients who do, many are not aware of the effects of their previous losses. In assessing patients, clinicians would be well advised to systematically consider the impact of losses and their relationship to presenting complaints.

ASSUMPTIONS ABOUT THE ROLE OF PSYCHOTHERAPY

Most people suffering from loss do not request, nor do they probably require, psychotherapy. However, if a clinician, when assessing a symptomatic patient, believes that internal conflictual obstacles to mourning are present, the option of psychotherapy should be considered. Psychotherapists have been trained to address aspects of loss that nonprofessional sources of support have not: for example, long-standing conflicts, maladaptive defenses, problem-generating behavior patterns, and factors contributing to low self-esteem. Among various treatment options, group approaches to psychotherapy have a number of advantages. These include reduction of social isolation and diminishment of the belief that one's difficulties are unique.

For a number of conceptual and economic reasons, short-term therapies are here to stay. Short-term group approaches are potentially among the most cost-effective forms of treatment. Time-limited therapy may be particularly appropriate for certain problems such as difficulty adjusting to loss. Patients are provided with the opportunity to reexperience loss and examine how they and others attempt to deal with it. However, short-term group therapy is not a panacea. Modest objectives such as diminishment of symptoms and a greater tolerance of ambivalent feelings toward the lost persons are certainly within its reach. In addition, short-term psychotherapy may help bring about more adaptive processes involving interpersonal relationships and productive performance in a variety of areas, long after the termination of therapy.

ASSUMPTIONS ABOUT CLINICAL RESEARCH

Despite recent reviews and claims about the general efficacy of psychotherapy, programs involving new combinations of techniques and patients, such as time-limited, short-term group therapy for loss patients, require controlled clinical trial evaluations. In addition to research questions concerning safety and efficacy, clinical trials can provide useful information about a number of related topics, for example, risk factors, selection criteria, natural remission of symptomatology, and process-outcome relationships. For the clinical setting, research inevitably introduces changes in customary procedures. It also creates certain constraints, and some contentious elements, such as, random allocation to conditions and multiple assessments. Nevertheless, clinical research and clinical practice can become well integrated and thereby serve both research and clinical objectives. To accomplish its goals, research must be well designed and involve a large sample of patients. In the past, investigators have greatly reduced their chances of obtaining significant results in clinical studies by studying small samples.

The assumptions that have been highlighted concerning the nature of loss, persons experiencing loss, the role of psychotherapy, and the importance of clinical research have all permeated and influenced the Short-Term Group Therapy Program for Loss Patients from its initial formative stages to the present time. Based upon our clinical experience in conducting over 25 such groups and our research experience in conducting a clinical investigation of 16 of those groups, we believe that a number of the assumptions have been confirmed, although others have admittedly not yet been tested. In the chapters that follow, we will attempt to highlight those hypotheses that we believe have received support, those that have not, and those that remain in need of empirical investigation.

CHAPTER **1**

The Extent of Person Losses and Associated Problems

Many writings that focus on loss begin by emphasizing its ubiquitous nature and the many negative experiences that
may follow its occurrence. For example, in his opening statement for
a series of articles concerning the biopsychosocial aspects of bereavement, Sidney Zisook (1987) stated:

> Grieving the death of a close friend or relative is an almost
> universal, potentially devastating experience that at some time
> or other affects us all. It is a prototypical life stress event which
> most often is associated with acute turmoil and distress, and,
> at times, may lead to substantial psychological and/or medical
> morbidity, possibly even to death. (p. xi)

Through the mass media we are constantly reminded of the
common occurrence of death. Yet, despite such repeated exposure,
and even though we accept the fact that death inevitably follows
life, we still experience as striking statistics that highlight the frequency of loss through death. The total number of people affected
is of course large. These statistics serve to highlight the fact that in
our everyday activities, whether leisure, love, or work, we continually interact with people who have recently experienced loss
through death and who may be suffering from its consequences. A
similar argument can be made about loss through divorce/separa-
tion from a partner. Again, the arts and media are filled with such
depictions. Nevertheless, and somewhat paradoxically, their very
commonality seems to make them less salient in our routine inter-

7

actions with people and may lead us to underestimate their presence and impact.

Patients referred to the Short-Term Group Therapy Program have experienced all types of person losses. Loss of a partner through death, that is, widowhood, and loss of a partner through divorce/separation are the most common. They are clearly among those losses most readily acknowledged as significant. Formal surveys have confirmed that loss of a partner through death or divorce/separation is considered to be one of life's most stressful events (Holmes & Rahe, 1967). Similarly, on Axis IV of the most recent *Diagnostic and Statistical Manual of Mental Disorders*, (DSM-III-R; American Psychiatric Association, 1987) the death of a spouse is defined as an extreme psychosocial stressor. Viewing the loss of a spouse in this way may partly explain why statistics concerning widowhood and divorce/separation are more plentiful and complete than those for other types of person losses. Closer examination of patients' histories reveals, however, that most have experienced a number of other types of such losses. These include loss of parents and loss of children during adulthood, and earlier events such as childhood parental loss and childhood sibling loss. Although a fair body of knowledge is available concerning the psychological impact of early traumatic events, statistical information lags behind that on adulthood losses.

LOSS THROUGH DEATH

In the case of widowhood, one of the best sources of information concerning its prevalence and potential negative consequences is the report from the study conducted by the Institute of Medicine of the National Academy of Sciences in the United States (Osterweis, Solomon, & Green, 1984). The statistics summarized in the report are frequently cited. It is estimated that 800,000 individuals become widows or widowers each year in the United States. This results in a prevalence figure of approximately 12 million persons. The ratio of women to men is 5:1. The statistics regarding widowhood are similar for Canada. In 1986 there were over 1¼ million widowed individuals (5% of the country's population). Of these, most (83%) were women. Although widowhood increases with age, 27% of the widows and 27% of the widowers were under age 65 (Statistics Canada, 1986). The statistics for widowhood are part of an aggregate in which, each year, 5–9% of the general population experience some form of bereavement. It has been estimated that as many as 800,000 parents lose a child through death each year in the U.S. (Osterweis et al., 1984).

One source of bereavement that has contributed to widowhood statistics as well as to other types, and which has created increasing concern, is death through violent acts. It has been noted that approximately 20,000 murders take place in the U.S. each year. A violent crime is said to occur every 24 seconds (U.S. Department of Justice, 1985). Public occurrences in community settings such as schools and restaurants have aroused media attention and created considerable alarm. In a recent article, Pynoos and Nader (1990) reviewed a number of forms of violence to which children are commonly exposed, and frequent negative consequences including posttraumatic stress symptoms. Crime can only serve to compound traumatization and hamper the mourning process in the survivors who indeed include many children as well as adult bystanders.

Osterweis et al. (1984) also documented the evidence of mortality and morbidity associated with conjugal bereavement. The authors cautioned the reader that the evidence is not as clear as once thought. They suggested that widowhood has an effect on mortality that is modified by gender. Young and middle-aged widowers are about 1½ times more likely to die prematurely than their married counterparts. The risk appears to continue for many years if the men do not remarry. The higher mortality rates are attributed to suicide, accidents, cardiovascular disease, and some infectious diseases that may result from immunological suppression following bereavement. In Canada, it has been estimated that two thirds of widowers are living under the poverty level (Statistics Canada, 1981). For widows in the U.S., there is some evidence suggesting increased mortality in the second year following bereavement, but not the first. For them, there is an increased risk of death from cirrhosis, presumably due to alcohol abuse, and perhaps from suicide.

Bereavement also appears to exacerbate and precipitate health-compromising behaviors. Increased use of alcohol, tobacco, tranquilizers, and other medicines is well documented among the bereaved, especially among people who had used such substances prior to their loss. Osterweis et al. (1984) further suggested that preexisting illness can be exacerbated. It has also been reported that some bereaved persons experience symptoms associated with the illness that killed the lost person (Zisook, Devaul, & Click, 1982). This phenomenon has been named "grief-related facsimile illness."

As to psychological morbidity, the immediate and short-term episodes of depression and anxiety are well known. Lindemann (1944) was among the first to document the phenomenology. More recently, Raphael (1983) has poignantly described the person's distress in the following way:

The absence of the dead person is everywhere palpable. The home and familiar environs seem full of painful reminders. Grief breaks over the bereaved in waves of distress. There is intense yearning, pining, and longing for the one who is dead. The bereaved feels empty inside, as though torn apart or as if the dead person had been torn out of his body. (p. 40)

There is less agreement among experts about the long-term nature of the bereavement reaction. What seems to be clear is that a definite proportion of the bereaved are diagnosably symptomatic after 1 year or more following their loss. In a series of studies published in the 1970s, Clayton and her colleagues (Bornstein, Clayton, Halikas, Maurice, & Robins, 1973; Clayton, 1973) assessed a group of 109 widows at various intervals after bereavement to assess the presence of depressive symptomatology. They found that 35% were depressed at 1 month and 17% at 1 year. A total of 47% were depressed at some time during the entire first year, compared with only 8% in a matched set of control subjects. In a more recent study involving 111 widows and widowers, Jacobs and Kim (1990) found an even higher percentage (27%) who were depressed after 1 year. In a second study, involving 102 widows and widowers, 13% met the criteria for panic disorder and 39% met the criteria for generalized anxiety disorder after 1 year. With regard to comorbidity, they reported that 56% of the bereaved spouses who had an anxiety disorder also suffered from major depression. These reports of prolonged psychiatric symptomatology are consistent with the conclusions of Zisook (1987), who has also studied the course of "unresolved grief." In his words, "grief did not simply end at six weeks, six months, or even six years. Although several features seemed to peak within one to two years, . . . many symptoms and behaviors continued to be present for years, perhaps indefinitely" (p. 27). In summary, there seems to be little doubt that bereavement has a number of sequelae that in various ways serve to increase morbidity and mortality rates for the bereaved.

LOSS THROUGH DIVORCE/SEPARATION FROM A PARTNER

Statistics on divorce are equally disturbing (Kirkpatrick, 1984). There has been a 700% increase in divorce since 1900 in the United States. One can compare the divorce rate relative to the population of 1915, which was 1:1,000, to that of 1966, which was 2.5:1,000, and to that of 1979, which was 5.3:1,000. The rate of increase is remarkable. It is also possible to compare divorce rates to marriage rates. Quoting U.S. statistics, Kirkpatrick wrote that in 1976, there were 50 divorces for every 100 marriages, and that Oregon and California led the list with 83 and 89 divorces, respectively, per 100 marriages. This pattern points to a possible future in which 50 of every 100 first marriages will result in divorce. She projects that, of those fifty, it is likely that 29 women will remarry and 13 will divorce again. Kirkpatrick (1984) also noted that divorce has replaced death as the most likely cause of marital dissolution according to a recent U.S. Census Report (1978).

Wallerstein (1986) conducted a 10-year longitudinal study of 60 divorcing families. Her findings point to a sobering reality, namely, that the losses incurred as a result of divorce are not within everyone's capacity to replace. Only 10% of the couples in the sample were able to make significant improvements in the quality of their lives following the divorce. In two thirds of the divorcing families, only one of the former spouses was able to do so. Those men and women who had initially opposed the divorce were found to be less likely to have improved the quality of their lives, compared with those former spouses who had initially sought divorce. For the women in the study, it was found that the capacity to rebuild both interpersonally and socioeconomically was age-related. Women in their 20s and 30s were found to be much more resilient following divorce than were those women who were forty or older at the time of divorce. It was also found that women who suffered from "severe neurotic problems" during their marriages were prone to subsequent impairment following divorce. Unresolved anger, especially in those women whose marriages prior to divorce were lengthy, seemed a persistent impediment to postdivorce health. Few people in the study seemed able to recognize their own contribution to the dissolution of the marriage. It is as if divorced people develop a blind spot in this area, regardless of how insightful they might be in any other. Divorce, for some, is a loss that seems more difficult than bereavement to work through. Failure to accept the loss, resolve the anger, and let go of the marriage point to interruptions in the mourning process following loss by divorce. The magnitude of the divorce rate can only be an indication that a vast second group of individuals are likely suffering losses they found themselves unable to deal with. This is highlighted by the fact that high-conflict families were excluded from the study. Therefore, none of the families were in litigation over custody or visitation rights at the time of the divorce. Furthermore, about half of all these women and men had been in brief or extended psychotherapy during the tenure of the study.

One cannot ignore the socioeconomic impact of divorce. Kirkpatrick (1984) reported that among the poor in the U.S., the single-mother family is the fastest growing population. She cites figures showing that two thirds of families entitled to child support are unable to collect. Furthermore, less than 5% of all divorced, nonremarried women are actually entitled to an alimony in a given year. Tragically, even fewer actually collect. In her opinion, this is tantamount to feminization of poverty that has been exacerbated, unexpectedly, by the legal system's reform leading to no-fault divorce laws. A 10-year study of the effects of this reform in California showed that the standard of living of the single-mother family decreased by 73%, whereas that of the man improved by 42% (Weitzman, 1985).

Benedek (1984) has summarized research and clinical evidence about the sequelae of divorce on children and adolescents as follows: To begin, in the nonpatient children of divorced families, long-term and lasting adverse reactions may occur. According to Benedek, the children of divorced families evidence more antisocial behavior, aggression, noncompliance, dependency, anxiety, depression, social difficulties, and problems in school. Brief supportive psychotherapy does not seem to be effective in preventing lasting effects. The adverse effects are also gender-related, as girls appear to be more severely affected. Benedek concluded that mental health professionals must be aware that a regular visitation pattern with a noncustodial parent is critical to the future mental health of the child.

It is important to recognize that any loss, especially for a child, is never experienced as a single loss but as a series of losses. Hence, the literature reveals that a child of divorce has to endure, among other possible effects, the total or partial yet permanent absence of one parent (usually the father); the acute and, it is hoped, temporary psychological loss of the other parent owing to preoccupation (usually the mother); the permanent loss of the family unit as the child had experienced it; and the temporary or permanent loss of the experience of a two-parent family. Such a variety of losses can lead to more than the acute grief and anxiety at the time of the divorce.

The emotional availability of one and both parents in the short and/or long term may be compromised and therefore could interfere with the child's developmental needs for identification, self-esteem regulation, formation of gender identity, and resolution of gender ambivalence. The existence of the non-in-house parent aggravates matters by encouraging the child's fantasies of parental reconciliation; behaviors and symptoms that arouse concern and hence the wished-for contact between both parents; confirmation of feelings of responsibility for the divorce when the quality, consistency, and/or predictability of visitations are lacking; and splitting the parental images into "all good" and "all bad" in response to the wishes of the in-house parent and the indulgence of the other parent. Perceiving the hated qualities of the non-in-house parent in the child, and consciously and unconsciously communicating the same to the minor, may set in motion a vicious circle of conflict between parent and offspring (Lohr & Chethik, 1990).

In summary, the foregoing review of studies outlines the demographics and effects of divorce on adults, adolescents, and children. Some of the authors believe that negative effects can be lessened, if not avoided, by more responsible parental behavior. That would include *not* withholding financial support, curtailing visitations, nor withdrawing from the children. Unfortunately, such reactions do occur frequently. The scope of the effects of these life events clearly reveals loss as a significant mental and physical problem.

CONCEPTUAL QUESTIONS

The material presented so far in this chapter has dealt with two epidemiologic questions. What is the incidence and prevalence of different types of person losses? What negative consequences are associated with different types of person losses? Independent of these questions are two conceptual questions that have proven considerably more difficult to answer, namely, What is the distinction between normal and abnormal reactions to loss? and What is the distinction between abnormal reactions to loss and certain types of psychiatric disorders?

With regard to the first question, most investigators have assumed that the distinction between normal and abnormal reactions is a valid one. A variety of terms have been used to denote abnormal reactions; these include pathologic grief, unresolved grief, morbid grief, complicated bereavement, and atypical bereavement. As with many other areas of classification in the mental health field, some have viewed the distinction as categorical and others as dimensional. Categorical proponents, who advocate distinct boundaries between classes, emphasize certain qualitative differences between normal and abnormal reactions to loss. It has been argued, for example, that strong ambivalence toward the lost person and low self-esteem are characteristic of abnormal not normal reactions to loss. This argument is consistent with Freud's (1917/1963) early differentiation between mourning and melancholia. Dimensional proponents, who advocate continuity between classes, emphasize certain quantitative differences between normal and abnormal reactions to loss. For example, some maintain that depressive symptoms such as sadness are more intense in the case of abnormal reactions, which is consistent with Clayton, Herjanic, and Murphy's (1972) position.

In a brief review article, Raphael and Middleton (1990) addressed the question, "What is pathologic grief?" They summarized distinguishing features that have been proposed by a number of workers in the field, attributing two important features to Bowlby (1980). One, which can be viewed as a qualitative difference, is the complete absence of conscious grieving. A variation of this feature is the complete absence of conscious grieving for a period of time followed by sudden onset, that is, a delayed reaction. Many therapists and theoreticians believe in the importance, even necessity, of openly grieving. The other feature, which can be viewed as a quantitative difference, is chronic mourning. In this case, aspects of the acute distressful reaction to loss persist for months or even years. One of the complicating factors in the effort to clarify the boundary between normal and abnormal reactions to loss, certainly in the case of duration, is the influence of culture. In a similar way, variation owing to individual differences such as age, religion, and personality has been noted. In their conclusion Raphael and Middleton argued that among the many features that have been proposed to distinguish pathologic from normal grief, the most frequently acknowledged are absence, delay, and chronicity of grief. To these three one can add a fourth, the debilitating impact of loss in terms of impaired functioning. This feature may be of particular importance for assessing the significance of cultural and individual differences.

Answers to the second conceptual question, which concerns the distinction between abnormal reactions to loss and certain types of psychiatric disorders, seem to have defied attempts to achieve consensus. A preliminary issue that has implications for the question is whether a grief reaction should ever be defined as a psychiatric disorder. The official position, represented by DSM-III-R (American Psychiatric Association, 1987), is that it should not. Only a V code category (conditions not attributable to a mental disorder) for "uncomplicated bereavement" is provided for a grief reaction, and it is said to rarely last longer than 3 months. Presumably, if significant symptoms persisted for longer than 3 months, they would have to be considered in terms of existing DSM-III-R disorders. Five disorders which some investigators have regarded as part of a pathologic grief reaction are depression (Clayton et al., 1972), posttraumatic stress disorder (Horowitz, 1990), hypochondriasis (Zisook, 1987), panic disorder, and generalized anxiety disorder (Jacobs & Kim, 1990).

The DSM-III-R position of not defining a grief reaction as a psychiatric disorder suggests that there is no distinction between abnormal reactions to loss and certain types of psychiatric disorders. A disadvantage associated with this position is that the impact of loss may be underestimated. By defining the abnormal manifestations of loss in terms of other psychiatric disorders, recognition of the contribution of loss is diminished. It should be remembered that DSM-III-R diagnoses are based almost entirely upon a consideration of symptomatology. Such diagnoses are also deliberately made with little or no consideration of etiology. Attempts to differentiate between abnormal reactions to loss and certain psychiatric disorders, for example, depression, upon the basis of symptomatology alone have proven unsuccessful. In contrast, if underlying etiologic factors are considered, distinctions can be made. Some of these distinctions will be considered in the following chapter, which concerns psychodynamically oriented theories about loss.

Perhaps in an effort to circumvent difficult conceptual questions, it has been argued that pathologic grief can simply be defined in terms of its consequences. If morbid outcomes like those described above follow loss, then the grief process is pathologic. The more morbid the outcome, the more pathologic the grief process is. Whereas this approach does allow one to avoid making questionable distinctions among normal reactions, abnormal reactions, and psychiatric disorders, it fails to provide an understanding of the pathogenesis of grief or a specification of the early signs of a pathologic process. This, in turn, may retard or preclude efforts to prevent a morbid outcome. To focus only upon consequences may also limit one's view and understanding. Clinicians who initially assess patients in mental health clinics routinely attempt to understand the meaning of the patient's complaints. By the time patients appear, symptomatology is usually well developed. If the patient's history reveals significant losses, a pathologic grief process may be suspected. More is needed, however, to make an accurate assessment of the problem and recommend appropriate treatment. A knowledge of risk factors and indicators that are independent of symptomatology is required. Such factors and indicators will be considered in Chapter 4. Many are theory-based, which is consistent with our belief that a solid conceptual basis facilitates accurate assessment of patients who have experienced loss.

CHAPTER 2

Psychoanalytic Theories of Pathologic Grief

Contributions from psychoanalytic writers have provided a unique vision and understanding of the phenomenon of loss. Whereas the psychoanalytic and object-relations theoretical understandings of loss primarily concern bereavement, the issues and processes involved in mourning any loss, be it by death or separation (divorce), are considered to be universal. This chapter reviews some of the theories of loss espoused by those writers.

In 1917, Freud introduced his thesis on "Mourning and Melancholia," with the warning that "the definition of melancholia is uncertain; it takes on various clinical forms (some of them suggesting somatic rather than psychogenic affections) that do not seem definitely to warrant reduction to a unity" (p. 152). Nevertheless, Freud (1917/1957a) did reduce the identification of melancholia, which we term pathologic grief, to a single feature. This notable feature that distinguished pathological from normal mourning processes was "a lowering of the self-regarding feelings to a degree that finds utterance in self-reproaches and self-reviling, and culminates in a delusional expectation of punishment" (p. 153). Otherwise, Freud considered the two processes to be the same: "a profoundly painful dejection, abrogation of interest in the outside world, loss of the capacity to love, [and] inhibition of all activity . . . " (p. 153).

The task of mourning involves accepting the reality that the relationship to the object (significant person) no longer exists. Hence, the emotional investment in or attachment to the lost object must be withdrawn. Freud (1917/1957a) noted that a struggle ensues between reality's dictate for withdrawal of "libido," or psychic energy, and the inertia of the previous investment of the same. In extreme cases, this struggle can lead to psychotic symptomatology, such as hallucinations of the deceased. In more typical cases, this struggle manifests itself as shock and denial. This period of shock and mourning is believed to be characteristic of the initial stage of bereavement and is further described in Chapter 3. To resolve the struggle and liberate the ego, a compromise is negotiated. "Each single one of the memories and hopes which bound the libido to the object is brought up and hypercathected, and the detachment of the libido from it accomplished" (Freud, 1917/1957a, p. 154). This process of detachment permits the continued existence of the lost object in the mind until the process is complete. The price of this continued existence is that the process of detachment is painful and gradual.

When a person resists accepting the significance or the impact of the loss such that the self-limiting process of mourning is arrested, pathologic grief is said to be occurring. Pathologic grief may appear as an absence of grief, as a prolonged mourning process, or as a grief reaction whose onset has been unusually delayed. Freud's (1917/1957a) contribution to understanding pathologic grief was his observation that, whereas normal mourning involves an attitude of loss of an object, pathologic grief involves an attitude of loss of self. Freud pursued his observation by focusing on the melancholic's self-criticisms. He noted that they were on moral rather than psychic grounds.

> The patient represents his ego to us as worthless, incapable of any effort and morally despicable; he reproaches himself, vilifies himself and expects to be cast out and chastised. He abases himself before everyone and commiserates his own relatives for being connected with someone so unworthy. (p. 155)

Freud noticed, however, an important contradiction. The melancholic was ironically shameless; proudly denouncing him- or herself for all to hear. "One could almost say that the opposite trait of insistent talking about himself predominates in the melancholiac" (p. 157). This contradiction was explained:

> If one listens patiently to the many and various self-accusations of the melancholiac, one cannot in the end avoid the impression that often the most violent of them are hardly at all applicable to the patient himself, but that with insignificant modifications they do fit someone else, some person whom the patient loves, has loved or ought to love. (p. 158)

According to Freud, the diminished self-esteem stems from the process of a narcissistic identification with the lost object. Reproaches against the self that diminish the self-esteem of the melancholic are understood as being originally directed at the lost, now introjected, object. The gradual, painful withdrawal of libido from the lost object does not occur in melancholia. Rather, the ego quickly abandons the lost object, thereby *identifying with* the abandoning, lost object.

> In this way the loss of the object became transformed into a loss in the ego, and the conflict between the ego and the loved person transformed into a cleavage between the criticizing faculty of the ego and the ego as altered by the identification. (p. 159)

It follows, therefore, that these reproaches reflect anger toward the lost object. Freud (1917/1957a) believed that the self-torments gratified sadistic tendencies and hatred towards the lost object. Hence, anger at the lost object predisposes the bereaved to develop melancholia (Zisook, 1987). Relationships characterized by such anger are considered highly ambivalent. Hence, the more the relationship with the lost object is characterized as ambivalent, the greater the likelihood of pathologic grief (Freud, 1917/1957a; Horowitz, Wilner, Marmar, & Krupnick, 1980; Lerner & Lerner, 1987; Tahka, 1984; Tyson, 1983).

Melanie Klein's (1948) contribution to the understanding of mourning is based on her elaboration of the works of Freud to include the primitive stages of development. She considered mourning to be an integral part of early age development leading to the "depressive position." Accordingly, under the influence of reality testing, the infant's ego gains in strength, evolving from the paranoid-schizoid position to that of the depressive. This evolution requires the perception that the bad and good objects are one and the same, a perception that heralds the attainment of ambivalence. The mother is experienced as giving and nurturing or "good," as well as unavailable and frustrating or "bad." In turn, this perception is coupled with the apprehension that the mother is the object of the child's fantasies and destructive impulses. Grieving over the loss of the good, loving, and nurturing past object is part of the depressive position. At the same time, the child experiences an actual loss through the process of weaning.

In adults, normal mourning activates early paranoid-schizoid and depressive anxieties. With the former anxieties, objects are again split into good and bad. Aggressive feelings are projected onto the lost object, followed by introjection. A process of feeling persecuted, leading to aggressive feelings towards the lost object, ensues. Furthermore, the mourner blames himself for the loss and experiences guilt. Only when the lost object is internalized as a whole object does the process of mourning culminate in a letting go (Bruch, 1989). Klein's (1948) work suggests that pathologic grief stems from the bereaved's inability to internalize the lost object as a whole object; the bereaved is unable to experience the lost object as being good and bad at the same time. In brief, it is the absence of ambivalence that characterizes pathologic grief. Therefore, those who fail to adequately negotiate the depressive position suffer a pathologic grief reaction in response to later bereavement.

Tahka (1984) discussed object loss from the viewpoint of personality development and object relatedness. He conceptualized the development of human personality as a function of coping with object loss through a developmental sequence of internalization methods. Tahka (1984) described three types of internalization processes. The first type was that of primary internalizations, which characterize the infant's earliest sensory impressions of his or her world. Through this process, the infant progressively gains experience in differentiating between inside and outside, self and other. Until the infant can differentiate between inside and outside, the concept of object relatedness, and, consequently, of object loss, is meaningless according to Tahka (1984).

The second type of internalization processes, introjection and identification, was considered the most important for the development of personality. Through introjection, inner objects or introjects are created to allow the infant to experience the object when he or she is absent. Introjects are representations of the other that are internal but do not belong to the self. They are, however, controlled by the self. They are created by the infant's subjective needs: an extension of the self that exists for the self. These introjects build and change the structures of the child's personality through identification with their different aspects and functions. For example, by identifying with the functions performed by the mother, now introjected, the child develops the capacity to perform the mothering functions for him- or herself. The extent to which the child can perform these functions for him- or herself is the extent to which the child is autonomous from the mother. Ultimately, the self develops the ability to perform all functions for which he or she once depended on external objects.

Relationships that are predominately characterized by the child's dependency on the object to perform need-gratifying functions are considered prestructural or functional. They are prestructural in that the object is experienced as "good" or "bad" depending on whether the subject's needs are being gratified or frustrated, respectively.

Hence, the object is split and "is not experienced as an individual human being, with motivations and characteristics of her own, but as a group of functions existing primarily for the child's sake (Tahka, 1984, p. 20)." The more the child identifies with the multitude of ego functions, the more the structure of his or her personality develops, and the more the child's prestructural relationships are transformed into poststructural ones. Poststructural relationships refer, therefore, to those whereby the child can appreciate the other person as an integrated whole with qualities that can gratify and frustrate the child while being independent of the child's needs.

Tahka (1984) posited that when a prestructural relationship is lost, the subject is faced with having to perform the function for him- or herself. Such an autonomous stance would necessitate a break from the prestructural object. Since the functional object is not experienced as distinct from the subject, a break from the object would be tantamount to a break from oneself. Such a break would threaten the subject with annihilation anxiety. Consequently, the object cannot be mourned but only replaced, insofar as the need must be serviced. This replacement may take the form of an immediate substitution of a new object, alcohol or drug abuse or both, psychosomatic symptoms, somatic disease, or depression. Hence, the more the object relatedness is characterized as prestructural, the greater the risk of pathologic grief.

The third type of internalization process, remembrance formation, referred to a mental process whereby the object becomes a conscious memory rather than an unconscious introject. Remembrance formation is similar to the gradual and painful process of decathecting posited by Freud (1917/1957a). Tahka (1984) described the process of mourning as involving two sequential reactions. First, an introject of the lost object is formed. This formation protects the subject from the unbearable experience of total object loss. The formation also guarantees an inner relationship for the working-through process to proceed. Next, the subject engages in a process of interaction and negotiation with this inner representation. According to Tahka, both prestructural and poststructural aspects of the relationship have to be addressed. Eventually, integration is achieved in that the introject is replaced by a conscious memory of the whole object. The subject interacts and negotiates with the introject until the object belongs to the past, where nothing more can be expected from it (Fenichel, 1945; Freud, 1917/1957a; Tahka, 1984).

Consistent with the work of Klein (1948), Tahka (1984) proposed that an individual was predisposed to pathologic grief when his or her relationships were characterized as prestructural. The subject cannot integrate the good and the bad aspects of the object into an ambivalently held, whole object. Freud (1914/1957b) referred to this type of object relationship as narcissistic: The object is not regarded as a separate entity but, rather, as part of the self and is used to serve a function that is normally internalized and carried out intrapsychically. However, he stopped short of linking this type of object relationship with melancholia: "The conclusion which our theory would require, namely, that the disposition to succumb to melancholia—or some part of it—lies in the narcissistic type of object-choice, unfortunately still lacks confirmation by investigation" (Freud, 1917/1957a, p. 160).

Many subsequent authors have linked the narcissistic object relations with melancholia. Forming that link is the reliance on an external object for self-esteem regulation. By tracing the development of self-esteem, it becomes clear why the formation of narcissistic object relations represents a predisposition for melancholia. Tyson (1983) linked positive self-esteem with the primary caretaker's (usually the mother) loving and concerned accessible presence, and with the pride with which she invests her child. If a loss, separation, or disappointment occurs prior to the establishment of internalized ideals, values, and self-worth, the subject will remain dependent on the presence of external objects to perform the praising and punishing functions. By failing to engender autonomy from her, the sustaining object, the mother fails to engender in her child the development of a constant sense of self and self-worth and leaves him or her forever vulnerable to pathologic grief (Tyson, 1983).

Lerner and Lerner (1987) agreed that the impact of loss covaries with the extent to which the psychic structures have been internalized and are autonomous from the sustaining object. Given that the lost object served a function for the person, the loss must be resisted (denied) until the function has been replaced. The person may deny the loss in the hope of completing the developmental process of separation and autonomy with the now introjected object. Similarly, Horowitz et al. (1980) posited that incomplete early separation from the mother figure rendered a person especially prone to pathologic grief. The intermediate step according to those authors, however, is the reemergence of troublesome, preexistent self-images and role relationship models. The sad response of the bereaved reflects a self-image of being a weak, abandoned, and needy waif. The angry response reflects a self-image of being a needy, evil, greedily consuming, destructive ogre. In both cases, the bereaved believe they have been left because of defects of the self. This belief leads to a feeling of deflation, shame, and dejection, accompanied by withdrawal or pathologic grief.

Bowlby (1963) approached the subject of mourning from the vantage point of motivation, adaptation, function, and object relations.

According to Bowlby, mourning is universally characterized by an initial stage of protest and an open expression of angry striving to retrieve the lost object. In infants, weeping serves the function of retrieving the mother. In children, reproaches serve the function of preventing future separations. In the bereaved, weeping and the open expression of sadness and of anger, coupled with the gradual acceptance of the permanence of the loss, all pave the way for a diminution of the attachment to the lost object. Bowlby disagreed with Freud that anger towards the deceased is diagnostic of pathologic grief. His first variant of pathologic grief posits that anger in reaction to loss is universally exhibited by infants, adults, and primates. His second variant states that it is the inability to accept and express this angry striving for the return of the lost object that characterizes pathologic mourning. Hence, Bowlby's view may be consistent with that of Klein. The inability to express both sadness and anger over the loss may reflect the inability to tolerate or experience ambivalence. When anger is prohibited, the bereaved remains preoccupied with thought and action directed at the lost object as if the object were still recoverable. In other words, the striving becomes repressed and unconscious and therefore not amenable to change. The unconscious yearning and displacement of anger are both understood as attempts at reunion with the lost object.

In cases of pathologic grief, the anger may be displaced onto the self or inappropriate objects. It is as though by maintaining the displacement, the bereaved is secretly and unconsciously awaiting the return of the lost object. When the anger is displaced onto the self, it is manifested as guilt. This guilt may reflect a sense of responsibility for the loss, including regret for past wishes that the object would go away. At times, the guilt may appear as totally irrational or of psychotic proportions, as in severe depressions. In extreme cases, the anger displaced onto the self may result in suicide.

Bowlby's third variant of pathologic grief is the caretaking of vicarious figures. In those cases, the bereaved disavows the loss, yearning, grief, helplessness, and anger. This disavowal is followed by a projection of these feelings onto others with similar misfortunes. In other words, projective identification is in operation. The bereaved identifies with the vicarious figure. He or she may also identify with the lost object and his or her family function. This proxy response is sometimes determined by social or familial pressures. For example, following the death of a mother, the oldest child may assume the caretaking role with the younger siblings.

A fourth variant of pathologic grief described by Bowlby includes the denial of the permanence of the loss. This denial continues despite a public acceptance of the reality of the loss. Therefore, although the loss is admitted, the permanence of the loss is denied. For example, during the early 1940s the Canadian prime minister, Mackenzie King, maintained through seances the fantasy of being in touch with his deceased mother. He never married, and his dog was his constant companion. The bereaved of this type tend to avoid therapy and all other close relationships, considering them a threat to the cherished secret.

Bowlby (1963) offered two predisposing conditions to the development of pathologic mourning. First, the relationship to the deceased was characterized as ambivalent because it was marred by hostile dependency, angry possessiveness, and insecure attachment. Second, this ambivalence had its roots in childhood bereavement over repeated separations and rejections. In summary, whereas Bowlby agreed that pathologic grief reflected relationships characterized by anger, he emphasized that it is the inability to express yearning and anger in response to loss rather than the anger per se that differentiates pathologic grief reactions from normal ones.

Worden (1982) translated the processes of mourning into four tasks and the phenomenon of pathologic grief into a failure to accomplish any of these four. The first task is to accept the reality of the loss and entails coming to believe that reunion with the deceased is impossible. Worden related the accomplishment of this task to Bowlby's initial stage of protest and open expression of angry striving to retrieve the lost object. Thus, Worden agreed with Bowlby that an initial denial of the fact, meaning, or irreversibility of the loss was normal and that only if this stage of "not believing" became protracted then the process was pathologic.

The second task of mourning, according to Worden, is to experience the pain associated with the loss. Again, consistent with Bowlby, Worden posited that the open expression of sadness and anger is a normal part of mourning, whereas the avoidance of the pain predisposes the mourner to pathologic grief. "Sooner or later, some of those who avoid all conscious grieving, break down—usually with some form of depression" (Bowlby, 1980, as cited in Worden, 1982, p. 14).

Worden's third task of mourning is to adjust to an environment in which the deceased is missing. When mourners fail to accomplish this task, they do not adapt to the loss. Rather, they promote their own helplessness. It is interesting to compare the writings of Tahka (1984), which we previously reviewed, with the following quote of Worden: "Many survivors resent having to develop new skills and to take on roles themselves that were formerly performed by their spouses" (Worden, 1982, pp. 14, 15). Hence, whereas Tahka (1984) emphasized the mourner's inability to perform the functions for him- or herself, Worden suggested that the mourner is unwilling to do so because of resentment.

The fourth task is to withdraw emotional energy and reinvest it in another relationship. This task is almost identical to Freud's characterization of the normal mourning process as "one of withdrawal of the libido from this [lost] object and transference of it to a new one" (Freud, 1917/1957a, p. 159). The failure to accomplish this task is reflected in the mourner "holding on to the past attachment rather than going on and forming new ones" (Worden, 1982, p. 16). Worden traced this failure to an avoidance of new relationships owing to a wish to avoid a repetition of the pain if another loss occurred, or guilt and disloyalty to the memory of the deceased. Although Worden acknowledged the difficulties of the four tasks of mourning, especially the fourth one, he emphasized that they can be successfully accomplished and that they are part of normal mourning.

Notwithstanding Bowlby's and Worden's observation that the human response to loss is universal, many authors have noted differences among the response of discrete populations. These populations include those who have lost a sibling in childhood, a parent in childhood, or a child. The following section summarizes characteristics of these populations that have been presented in the literature.

CHILDHOOD SIBLING LOSS

Because a sibling is not as crucial as a parent for a child's development, childhood sibling loss is more likely to be traumatic than tragic. However, the impact of the loss is contingent on the parents' capacity to adequately negotiate their own mourning process while remaining emotionally available for the surviving sibling(s). Their emotional availability should ideally include their facilitation of the grieving process for the remaining youngsters. The parents who fail to successfully mourn the death of their child will concurrently impede the mourning process for their surviving children (Pollock, 1989). These impediments may result from the parents resorting to denial, physical or emotional withdrawal, idealization of the dead child, overprotection and control of the surviving children, or treating a remaining child as a replacement for the dead one.

Many authors (Chapman, 1959; Freud, 1916/1963, 1917/1957a; Hilgard, 1969) have emphasized the role of survivor guilt when a sibling dies. Survivor guilt refers to the sense of feeling unentitled to live because the other has died. Such guilt has been attributed to early sibling rivalry. It may also mirror the parents' own guilt regarding their failure to prevent the loss. The parents' guilt may result, therefore, in a shift in their sense of self from one where strength, concern, and worthiness are present to images of weakness, incompetence, and lack of compassion (Horowitz et al., 1980). This self-image may be projected onto the surviving children. This projection colludes with the siblings' survivor guilt by consciously or unconsciously holding the remaining children responsible for the loss. The popular movie of a few years ago, *Ordinary People* (Schwary & Redford, 1980) poignantly depicted such a situation. The surviving child became full of despair and suicidal in reaction to his mother's silent accusations. Moreover, her accusations were interpreted by the son as her wish that he had died and that his brother had survived. On occasion, the remaining child may indeed have been responsible for the sibling's death. Such a situation was depicted in the movie *Stone Boy* (Bloch, Roth, & Cain, 1984). In that film, a young boy accidentally shot his brother. The parents, paralyzed by their grief, ostracize their young son. The popularity of these films suggests that their relevance may exceed the experience of sibling loss. Survivor guilt is a pervasive experience that may follow any loss. The guilt may also reflect the survivor's celebration of his or her continued life. According to Pollock (1989):

> in talented individuals, the death of a sibling can stimulate or direct creativity. The creative product can show evidence of the sibling-loss event, the type of mourning process utilized and, at times, it becomes a restitutional or reparational product to replace the lost object. Loss however does not account for the creative potential.

Although Pollock offered his description of some creative subjects to reflect a positive adaptation to sibling loss, the agony and despair of the subjects permeates the descriptions. One cannot but wonder whether any of them had been truly liberated through their art.

CHILDHOOD PARENTAL LOSS

Childhood parental death is perhaps one of the most tragic losses. The long-term consequences are difficult to ascertain because they are contingent on several mediating variables. These variables are considered risk factors and are presented in Chapter 4. The intermediate impact of early bereavement is the greater likelihood of an adolescence characterized by depression, school dysfunction, and delinquency

(Krupnick & Solomon, 1987). The impact of childhood parental death reflects its multiple ramifications. These include financial burdens, additional domestic responsibilities, the temporary psychological loss of the surviving parent, and the permanent loss of the family unit. Furthermore, the psychological immaturity of the child renders him or her more vulnerable to psychopathology in the short, intermediate, and long term. Common reactions among children to parental loss have been discerned (Bloom-Feshbach, Bloom-Feshbach, & Associates, 1987; Dietrich & Shabad, 1990; Pollock, 1989). These reactions have been compared (Bowlby, 1960) and contrasted (Wolfenstein, 1966) with adults' reactions to loss. It seems prudent to expect individual variation as well as commonalities among children in their reaction to parental death. Furthermore, it is also expected that children's response to death reflects developmental milestones, for example, object constancy. Hence, the very young's seeming lack of response, absorption in play, or announcing the death of the parent(s) "inappropriately" can be understood as attempts to master this most traumatic event in a way that is consistent with their level of maturity (Krupnick & Solomon, 1987). Given their lack of maturity, however, the mourning process may rapidly become impeded. This impediment renders children at risk of denying the loss or of developing a manifest grief later in life, or both. Conversely, the response of older children would presumably approximate the adult reaction to death such that they are better equipped to resolve the mourning process.

Krupnick and Solomon (1987) noted that particular risk factors for pathologic grief include loss before the age of 5 years or during early adolescence, loss of the mother for girls under age eleven, and loss of the father for adolescent boys. These identified risk factors may reflect vulnerabilities associated with particular developmental stages. Losing a parent during the preoedipal period is disruptive for boys and girls alike. It would seem, however, that adolescence is a crucial time for boys to identify with father, whereas latency is a crucial time for girls to identify with mother. These differences are consistent with the common belief that girls tend to reach psychosocial maturity sooner than boys.

One common theme in terms of childhood parental loss is highlighted by Dietrich (1989) under the rubric of the "lost immortal parental complex." He explained:

> Here the lost, dead parent is immortalized in a core: an organized constellation of unconscious fantasies and is reflected in various facets of object relations, self and object representations, in identification, introjects, incorporated objects, as well

as in preconscious and conscious longings, wishes and fantasies.

The complex has many aspects. One aspect concerns the child's fantasy that he or she destroyed the parent. This fantasy is believed to stem from the aggressive impulses and hostile wishes that a child typically holds for a parent. The fantasy evokes guilt that also becomes part of the lost–immortal parent complex. The guilt is particularly potent if the parent who died was of the same sex as the child. In such cases, the guilt is associated with an actual oedipal victory. In this respect it is interesting to note that an identified risk factor for future difficulties is an emotionally vulnerable surviving parent who becomes overly dependent on the child (Krupnick & Solomon, 1987). Perhaps the parent's dependency, misinterpreted as intimacy, exacerbates the child's guilt over oedipal victory.

An oedipal union is also fantasied, however, if the parent who died was of the opposite sex. In those cases, the child idealizes him or her (Fenichel, 1953) and experiences the parent as his or her "very own." Dietrich believed that the fantasy that the dead parent has become the bereaved's "very own" is potent and central to the complex. This particular fantasy can occur regardless of which parent dies. Its appeal is derived from its ability to permit an ongoing relationship with the dead parent. The fantasy restores the parent to the child as if to say "I'm not finished with you yet." In the fantasy, however, the child has control over the parent's activities rather than being the helpless recipient of the whims of either the parent or fate. Unlike the memory of the parent, the fantasized parent is forever available to the child. This availability that the fantasy offers seems to compensate for all that it cannot provide the child. In some ways it is preferable for the introject to be always sadistic, for example, than unpredictable, uncontrollable, and able to render the child feeling helpless (Tahka, 1984).

Other authors alluding to the above complex hold the proposition that some bereaved children might feel guilty enough to fear the return of the deceased parent(s) to exact retribution, or that fate may demand that they succumb to a similar demise (Arthur & Kemme, 1964). Conversely, Furman (1974) suggested that self-blame may serve a defensive function in that the passive helplessness of bereavement is transformed into an active responsibility. Another constellation in bereaved children centers around the fantasy that the death of the parent(s) was an act of desertion. The belief that the parents abandoned the child can undermine his or her self-esteem. The child may feel unlikeable, unlovable, and unworthy. He or she may also feel physically small and emotionally helpless (Call & Wolfenstein, 1976). It is as if the child believes that the parent left because of defects in the child (Horowitz et al., 1980).

CHILD LOSS

Perhaps the fate of some parents, particularly mothers, who lose a child during their lifetime is as tragic as childhood parental loss. It is not uncommon for parents across cultures to consider dying before one's offspring as a blessing. With the tendency in the industrialized countries to enjoy low infant mortality rates, the death of a child is becoming even less and less expected. For some parents, again especially mothers, the effect of the death of a child might be a particularly protracted grieving period. In some cases, the grief may never be resolved. Freud expressed his own personal grief over the sudden death of his 27-year-old daughter "dear blooming Sophie" Halberstadt. To Ferenczi he wrote:

> Since I am the deepest of unbelievers, I have no one to accuse and know that there is no place where one can lodge an accusation . . . way deep down I sense a feeling of a deep narcissistic injury I shall not get over." (Gay, 1988, p. 393)

Nine years later, on the anniversary of Sophie's 36th birthday, he wrote to his lifelong friend, the Swiss psychiatrist, Binswanger:

> We know that the acute grief we feel after the loss will come to an end, but that we will remain inconsolable, and will never find a substitute. Everything that comes to take place of the lost object, even if it fills it completely, nevertheless remains something different. (cited in Pollock, 1989, p. 29)

According to Rubin (1984):

> Resolution implies that the bereaved should neither overidealize nor denigrate and devalue the deceased. The lost other should be neither too close nor too distant from the active self-representations, and neither overpower nor be overpowered by the self-representations. (p. 343)

Shucter and Zisook (1987) wrote that if acceptance means that the bereaved truly experience that the relationship with the lost object is over, finished, and done with, then it is an extraordinary person who achieves acceptance. The impact of anniversary reactions testifies to the lifelong effect of loss. Hence, one can wonder whether a mourning process is ever pathologic if it can be lifelong. The next chapter considers the different kinds of resources that are available to persons who are suffering from loss.

CHAPTER **3**

Available Resources for Those Who Have Suffered Person Losses

In a concluding statement from their chapter on bereavement intervention programs, Osterweis, Solomon, and Green (1984) identified the main sources of support for the bereaved.

> The evidence suggests that everyone needs support, reassurance, and some education and information following bereavement. This may be provided by family, friends, or clergy in an informal way, by laypeople in similar circumstances, by a community support group, or by health professionals. (pp. 272–273)

Although each of these sources is a potential provider of support, evidence suggests that opportunities for receiving help from traditional sources such as family and friends have been decreasing during the present century, and that service from frontline health providers such as physicians and nurses has been uneven. Consequently, responsibility for providing support, especially sustained support, has shifted to community groups. Decreased opportunities for traditional support may also have contributed to an increase in the incidence of abnormal reactions to loss, and consequently to the number of patients coming to the attention of mental health professionals.

This chapter will focus on several related topics. First, societal changes in the availability of support for the bereaved will be considered. Second, a framework for organizing services provided by both lay and professional persons will be presented. Third, individual interventions will be summarized; and fourth, group interventions will be reviewed.

SOCIETAL CHANGES

Society has a role to play in the drama surrounding the loss of one of its members, as does the family in recalling the mourner to his place among the living. Yet society's relationship to the mourner has always been as ambivalent as that of the mourner to himself and to his lost object. The mourner, after all, reminds us of whom he has lost, that death has come to visit, and that our own life is also vulnerable. We do not like to be reminded, states Freud (1915/1957c), that "everyone owes nature a death and must expect to pay the debt" (p. 289).

Freud recognized that there can be no mental representation for death, because it is simply a negation, that is, the absence of what we know as life. All symbols of death, however florid, are mere transpositions of living images by which we seek to fill a void in our imagination, a void that has to do with the ultimate loss of our own existence. According to Freud (1915/1957c), "Our unconscious, then, does not believe in its own death; it behaves as if it were immortal. What we call our unconscious, the deepest strata of our minds made up of instinctual impulses, knows nothing that is negative, and no negation; in it [contradictions] coincide. For that reason it does not know its own death, for to that we can give only a negative content" (p. 296).

It has always been common to find people who believe that death is a way out of life's difficulties. It has usually been imagined as a state of sleep or repose, a haven from pain, suffering, and fear. It is not difficult to empathize with such wishes. Today, however, many people seem to have adopted a more extreme position; they profess that the death that they seek is nothingness. They have no representation for it and do not seem to desire one. Ariès (1982), in his book *The Hour of Our Death*, regards this outlook as characteristic of a new culture. He charts how the idea of death has evolved in our culture since classical and medieval times and identifies the symbols representing death in art and literature, as well as in funerary and burial customs. Ariès maintains that symbols of death are no longer prominent in the new culture, and that gone with them is a link to the past that in previous generations provided meaning and a sense of continuity for the living. In his terms, "the change consists precisely in banishing from the sight of the public not only death but with it, its icon. Relegated to the secret, private space of the home or the anonymity of the hospital, *death no longer makes any sign* "(italics his) (p. 266).

It was generally believed, whether true or not, that the sites of many hospitals were selected because they were close to graveyards. This may have reflected nineteenth-century popular wisdom that the hospital was a place where you go to die. The widening role of the hospital in general medical care has not changed this, however much the acceptance of this fact has diminished. The hospital is now seen as standing between the patient and death. Death in the hospital is, by nineteenth-century standards, dehumanized. The patient is often lost in the life-preserving machine and may become, for those caring for him, a preparation, a substrate upon which to practice, by rote, meaningless (even if technologically correct) medical acts. The emphasis is on clinging to life at the expense of preparing for death.

People react to death as though it were an affront or a mistake. They hold the doctor responsible, and he is the repository of both their magical wish for immortality and of their anger and frustration when confronted with death. Resuscitation may become a performance the outcome of which is a measure of personal success or failure for the physician. The loss of a patient through death may then be a blow to the physician's narcissism, and his self-esteem may be further diminished by the irate family's critical attitude. Survivors in the early phase of shock, before grief is internalized, project angry feelings, which originate in ambivalence towards the lost loved one, onto caretakers, whom they blame for having been incompetent, negligent, and sloppy in their ministrations to the deceased (Freud, 1917/1957a). This often engenders anxiety and guilt in the caretaker, whose first concern may be to defensively cover his tracks, reassuring himself that he has done everything humanly possible, and spending time obsessively checking that he has not made a mistake for which he can be sued. This withdrawal and mutual distrust between caretaker and survivor is the result of the primitive, unreasonable, and largely unconscious wish (shared by both) to deny death its proper place in the lexicon of the living.

Religion and its institutions have always played an important part in consoling the mourner and providing a structure within which grief might be contained. In the past two centuries, however, religious institutions have gradually ceded this role to more secular organizations. One may well ask, Where in society today is one encouraged to speak about loss and grief? The funeral is brief. There is little time for lingering customs such as the Irish wake or the Jewish *shiva*. There is little time for mourning. Society's attitude is exemplified by statements like "He died in his sleep," "He just didn't wake up," "It was the best possible way to go" (Ariès, 1985, p. 587). These encourage denial and do not allow for mourning. The dead seem to be cast aside and with them the process of mourning.

Even in circumstances where funerary customs are preserved, societal pressure "to get on with one's life" may severely restrict the mourning process. In the case of the following patient, the death of a friend's wife reawakened concerns about the place of death in his life.

> When my father died, my mother just kept on going. She taught, worked on her festival, looked after my grandmother for 4 years until her death, and then she was free. She traveled a bit after that. She certainly did not go off the deep end and she was a model for me. Death is such an interesting thing. There was Uncle Perry and my dad: brief sicknesses, then people just carried on. There was never a falling apart after death. It was just a part of living. They just had a wake and a funeral. People went on just as well after they lost a spouse. The Catholic custom was that the body was brought over to the house, people came over, and tea was served. I must have been to a dozen wakes. The only one that hit me was my father's. The others were like going for a visit.

Except for his father's death, the others, as Ariès described, seemed to make no "sign." The consequence for the patient was that he felt compelled to give up ties with his past that would have given depth and meaning to his present life. He rarely contacted his two living sisters, and he had an estranged brother from whom he had not heard in 5 years and for all he knew might even be dead. He was profoundly unhappy with himself and had sought therapy to express grief and do the work of mourning.

In a second case, a boy of 10 was shielded from the grief of his parents by being sent to relatives during the acute mourning period after the death of his 6-year-old brother. Every year the Christmas season would arouse a deep and inexplicable feeling of sadness in him. His brother, with whom he had been very close, had died in a vehicle accident on Christmas Eve. The parents, who had failed to resolve their own grief, never mentioned the lost sibling, and his pictures and personal effects (which aroused painful memories) were hidden away. Twenty-five years later, in therapy, the patient explored his sad feelings, and his associations led back to his brother. He searched for and found the neglected grave and for the first time was able to mourn openly. Many repressed memories and feelings returned, with a concomitant increase of self-esteem and a lessening of depression. Each year the mourner returns to the grave, permitting continued reexpression and working through of mourning.

There is evident conflict today between society's wish to deny death and the more rational belief held by the scientific community that mourning is an essential human condition. Ariès points that out:

> Society avoids [widowers] whether they are young or old, but
> especially if they are old, . . . They have no one to talk to about
> the only subject that matters to them, the person they have lost.
> There is nothing left for them to do but die themselves, and that
> is often what they do, without necessarily committing suicide.
> (p. 583)

This last point is supported by the literature concerning increased mortality and morbidity following the loss of a significant other.

If, as it has been noted, today "death and mourning are treated with the same prudery as the sexual impulses were a century ago" (Gorer, 1965, p. 579), then we are faced with the same task with regard to mourning as Freud was with regard to sex in Victorian times. Ariès points out that "society regards mourning as morbid, whereas for the psychologists it is the repression of mourning that is pathological."

Osterweis et al. (1984) also link societal changes to decreased opportunities for mourning. They highlight the decline of kinship and religion, nuclearization of the family, high mobility, diminished sense of community, and disengagement of the elderly as contributing factors in Western society. They point out that most deaths occur in hospitals and nursing homes. Thus institutions have removed death from the home and concealed many aspects of death and dying. Because grief is no longer shared and ritualized, there is uncertainty about the place of mourning. The underlying message, though, is clear. Mourning should be brief and private. This message is reinforced by the limited time allotted to the funeral and to the period of mourning before one is expected to return to work and/or other regular activities.

Osterweis et al. also consider the various aspects of social support that are thought to facilitate the grief process and recovery from bereavement. They include enhancing self-esteem and feeling loved, problem solving, networking, and providing relationship resources for making life-style transitions. It is hard to imagine how sufficient support can be obtained from family and friends when there are such strong societal pressures to limit the mourning process. Considering the institutional location of most deaths, one would expect that substantial pressure to provide support is directed toward health professionals who are at the scene of death, for example, physicians and nurses. Whereas health professionals are able to provide sufficient support in some circumstances, the reality of busy ward schedules, minimal training, mixed feelings about the circumstances of death (e.g., feeling guilty *and* feeling satisfied that every avenue was tried) and disinclination to serve as a grief counselor in the absence of direct reimbursement suggests that they often do not. Given these circumstances and the general societal changes highlighted in this section, it is not surprising that a number of self-help and mutual-help community groups have arisen to fill the void. Before we consider such groups, as well as the forms of intervention that tend to be provided by traditional mental health professionals, an organizational framework will be offered to facilitate the review.

CONCEPTUAL FRAMEWORK

Reactions to loss can be classified according to two independent dimensions. The first is stage of mourning (initial vs. transitional), and the second is type of mourning (normal vs. abnormal). All reactions to loss involve painful experiences that can be frightening to the bereaved and to those with whom they interact. Typically, a number of demands are placed upon those surrounding the bereaved. One type of response to normal reactions to loss is counseling, which generally involves supportive techniques. Its objective is to assist the client in progressing through the normal stages of mourning. In contrast, a response to abnormal reactions to loss is therapy, which may involve interpretive techniques. Its objective is to assist the patient in removing obstacles to progressing through the normal stages of mourning. Other responses, for example, the provision of medication, are available and will also be considered below.

With regard to stage, mourning reflects a progression from an initial period of shock and grief to a period of coping with life-style changes evoked by the loss. The distinction between initial versus transitional stages of loss has been clarified by investigators who have conceptualized the mourning process as consisting of a number of tasks. Of these, Worden (1982) identified four. They include (1) acceptance of the reality of the loss, (2) experience of the pain of grief, (3) adjustment to an environment in which the deceased is missing, and (4) withdrawal of emotional energy and reinvestment in another relationship. The first two tasks can be associated with the initial stage, and the last two tasks can be associated with the transitional stage. In a similar vein, Zisook (1987) differentiated six major tasks. They include (1) development of the capacity to experience, express, and integrate painful affects; (2) utilization of the most adaptive means of modulating painful affects; (3) integration of the continuing relationship with the dead spouse; (4) maintenance of health and continued functioning; (5) achievement of a successful reconfiguration of altered relationships; and (6) achievement of an integrated, healthy self-concept and a stable world view. Again, the first two tasks can be associated with the initial stage and the remaining tasks with the transitional stage.

With regard to the type of mourning, most investigators have assumed that the distinction between normal and abnormal reactions is a valid one. As indicated above, however, the boundary between the two has often been unclear. In Chapter 1 several features were identified as characteristic of abnormal reactions. They include the absence of grief, delayed grief, prolonged grief, and the presence of diagnosable psychiatric disorders. Extreme reactions are obviously more readily classified as abnormal.

During the initial stage, survivors who are experiencing a normal mourning process typically do not seek help outside their immediate social network. They depend upon the support of family, friends, and religious acquaintances. After several weeks, however, attention usually wanes as significant others return to their customary social routines. At this time, the onset of the transitional stage, the real impact of the loss may begin to be felt. The survivor is expected to get on with his or her life, which for most people means taking on new life-styles and new responsibilities, some of which previously belonged to the lost persons. Questions concerning competence and self-esteem come to the fore. It is at this point that some survivors seek the assistance of outsiders, particularly those who have had similar experiences in making life-style transitions following loss. Much of what is needed and provided consists of support, information, and help in solving everyday problems. The objective is to assist the person in progressing through the various tasks (and stages) of mourning. This type of assistance can be defined as grief counseling.

Abnormal reactions to loss, which involve forms of overreaction or underreaction, have elicited different types of intervention. Overreaction during the initial stage has typically been treated with medication. Anxiety and agitation have prompted the prescription of antianxiety drugs such as minor tranquilizers. The presence of insomnia has prompted treatment with hypnotic drugs. Less frequently, signs of depression have been treated with antidepressant drugs. Clinicians who prescribe such medications often do so reluctantly. Risks of drug dependence, suicidal behavior, and lethal reactions if the drugs are combined with alcohol are prominent. In addition, their use runs counter to the notion that a painful grief reaction is normal and should be allowed to run its course. As Osterweis et al. (1984) pointed out, the prescription of drugs during the initial stage of mourning operates entirely without the validation of controlled, clinical trial studies.

Underreaction during the initial stage has prompted the use of several psychosocial techniques, usually with a behavioral orientation, designed to expose the bereaved to painful stimuli associated with the loss. Some of the techniques are described in the following section on individual interventions. These, like a variety of psychosocial techniques offered during the transitional stage, attempt to remove obstacles to completing the tasks (and stages) of mourning. Thus they can be defined as a form of grief therapy. In general, therapy has tended to address the needs of those experiencing abnormal (pathologic) mourning processes, whereas counseling has tended to address the concerns of those experiencing normal mourning processes. Exceptions to this pattern do exist. It should be emphasized that some forms of therapy and counseling share common features. These include providing support, facilitating and managing grief, and developing or modifying coping skills. Another feature that serves to distinguish various psychosocial techniques is whether they are provided individually or within a group. The next two sections are organized according to this feature.

INDIVIDUAL INTERVENTION METHODS

In general, difficulties during the initial stage of mourning, which tend to involve denial of the loss and, consequently, denial of the painful affects associated with it, have been addressed by individual intervention methods. The various methods and the investigators who have described them are listed in Table 3.1. Crisis intervention and supportive problem-solving techniques have been commonly used. In addition to crisis intervention, Raphael (1983) has also used interpretive techniques. Melges and DeMaso (1980) have used a cognitive "regrief" approach that emphasizes guided imagery for reliving, revising, and revisiting scenes of the loss, for example, the funeral. Ramsey (1977) has used the behavioral techniques of flooding and prolonged exposure to stimuli associated with the loss. Volkan (1975) has used an approach that includes identifying linking objects, in other words, reminders which link the person to the deceased, emotionally reliving the circumstances of the death, and visiting the grave site. The interpretive part of Raphael's approach and the approaches of Melges and DeMaso, Ramsey, and Volkan constitute therapy because they are aimed at identifying and removing obstacles to the mourning process with patient populations.

An individual therapy method that addresses issues associated with both the initial and transitional stages was described by Horowitz, Marmar, Weiss, DeWitt, and Rosenbaum (1984). It is a time-limited psychodynamic approach. The objective is to identify and re-

TABLE 3.1. Individual Intervention Methods and Investigators Categorized by Stage of Mourning (Initial, Transitional) and Type of Service (Counseling, Therapy)

Initial stage—counseling	*Investigator(s)*
Crisis intervention/supportive problem solving	Raphael (1983)
Initial stage—therapy	
Identification of linking objects	Volkan (1975)
Flooding/prolonged exposure to stimuli	Ramsey (1977)
Cognitive regrief through guided imagery	Melges & DeMaso (1980)
Interpretive therapy	Raphael (1983)
Initial & transitional stages—counseling	
Widow-to-Widow Program	Silverman (1969)
Grief counseling	Worden (1982)
Initial & transitional stages—therapy	
Individual therapy	Worden (1982)
Time-limited dynamic psychotherapy	Horowitz et al. (1984)
Interpersonal therapy	Klerman et al. (1984)

Note. Tasks associated with the initial stage include accepting the loss and experiencing painful affects. Tasks associated with the transitional stage include adjusting to the environment and reinvesting energy in new relationships. Counseling assists the person in progressing through the stages of mourning. Therapy assists the person in removing obstacles to mourning processes.

solve conflicts (obstacles) related to the mourning process and maladaptive relationship patterns. Themes activated by the loss are explored by means of catharsis; confrontation of current resistances; and interpretation of defensive styles, warded-off ideas, and repressed emotions. An individual therapy method that was developed to treat depression, including that which is part of an abnormal grief reaction, is the interpersonal therapy of Klerman, Weissman, Rounsaville, and Chevron (1984). This approach is focused and time limited. It attends to current symptoms and their interpersonal context and attempts to free the patient from a maladaptive attachment to the lost person. In contrast to psychodynamic therapy, it does not focus on internal unconscious components of intrapsychic conflict. Another individual therapy method for pathologic grief was outlined by Worden (1982). Its goal is to identify and resolve the conflicts of separation that preclude the completion of mourning tasks.

Worden advocated a variety of techniques to serve this purpose, including the Gestalt "empty chair" method, role-playing psycho-drama, focusing on "linking objects," and more traditional forms of interpretation.

Worden (1982) also outlined techniques associated with grief counseling, whose goal is the more modest one of helping people who are experiencing normal grief reactions to complete the various tasks of mourning within a reasonable time. Similar in purpose, and there-fore a form of counseling, is the Widow-to-Widow Program of Phyllis Silverman (1969). This program, one of a number of well-organized self-help and mutual-help programs, is based on the assumption that someone who has experienced and adapted well to loss is potentially an ideal caregiver for the bereaved. The program has followed a public-health, preventive approach. Recently (3–6 weeks)—but not immediately—bereaved widows are personally contacted by another widow with an offer of assistance and friendship. Help in finding a job, sorting out finances, and rearing children is commonly provided. The program grew from an initial pilot project in the Boston area to a national and international network. Like the therapy approaches ear-lier described, this counseling approach advocates individual rather than group contacts at the initial stage. The widows are regarded as nonreceptive to group counseling until several months after their losses. This conclusion was also formed by Rogers, Vachon, Lyall, Sheldon, and Freeman (1980).

GROUP INTERVENTION METHODS

As indicated in Table 3.2, group intervention methods have addressed the transitional stage of mourning. The absence of group intervention methods at the initial stage seems to suggest that caregivers believe it premature to use a group format to treat pathologic mourners who are impeded at this time. Almost all of the group intervention methods have emphasized support and education as a means of helping per-sons deal with the tasks of mourning. Most group participants can be regarded as experiencing normal, as opposed to abnormal, reactions to grief. The fact that many of the participants were volunteer recruits from the community rather than patients who presented at a mental health clinic is consistent with this viewpoint. We wish to emphasize here that the designation of most group interventions as counseling is not intended to discount or minimize the importance or contributions of these secondary prevention methods, especially given the high-risk status of the bereaved. As many of the reports indicate, the use of the

TABLE 3.2. Group Intervention Methods and Investigators Categorized by
Stage of Mourning (Initial, Transitional) and Type of Service (Counseling,
Therapy)

Transitional stage—counseling	Investigator(s)
Self-help, confidant, and consciousness raising groups	Barrett (1978)
Widow-to-widow groups	Vachon et al. (1980)
Self-help, cognitive restructuring, and behavioral skills groups	Walls & Meyers (1985)
THEOS self-help groups	Lieberman & Videka-Sherman (1986)
Mutual-help groups	Marmar et al. (1988)
Support groups	Yalom & Vinogradov (1988)
Transitional stage—therapy	
Short-term group psychotherapy	McCallum & Piper (1988)

Note. There are no methods for the initial stage.

services of paraprofessionals to implement those methods is an efficient strategy.

A number of group intervention methods have been used in
formal studies that were designed to evaluate their effectiveness. The
findings from those studies and their implications will be reviewed in
Chapter 7. Reference to group methods in the present chapter is part
of an effort to provide as complete an overview as possible of the
different kinds of group intervention methods described in the literature. One such type of group intervention that used the principles of
the Widow-to-Widow Program has been set up to follow initial one-
to-one contact (Vachon, Lyall, Rogers, Freedman-Letofsky, & Freeman,
1980). The subsequent "small group meetings" were set up to discuss
mutual concerns among the widows. Support, practical assistance,
and friendship were provided by the members of the groups as they
had been by the individual widow caregivers. Rogers, Vachon, Lyall,
Sheldon, and Freeman (1980) reported that over time, widows in this
program came to prefer larger, more structured groups with focused
discussions about vocational and social problems. Another supportive
group approach was provided by the international self-help organization known as THEOS (They Help Each Other Spiritually). A variety
of group meetings with educational, social, and supportive functions
were sponsored (Lieberman & Videka-Sherman, 1986). Characteristic
of the Widow-to-Widow and THEOS programs is that the contacts

with widows and widowers were not time limited. They were available for as long as they were needed.

In contrast to the open-ended group meetings described above, a number of time-limited, short-term group interventions for widows, which were part of evaluative studies, have been described in two publications. Three types of support groups, each consisting of seven once-weekly 2-hour sessions were studied by Barrett (1978). As she described: (1) The purpose of the "self-help" groups was to encourage participants to help each other find solutions to the problems of widowhood. Such problems included loneliness, single parenting, finances, employment, legal issues, and relationships with men. (2) The purpose of the "confidant" groups was the development of close friendship between pairs of widows. Intimacy-building tasks were conducted in the groups. (3) The purpose of the "consciousness raising" groups was to facilitate the participants' awareness of how their experiences as widows concerned them as women. At each session specific sex-role topics were chosen and discussed. Thus the overall approach taken by Barrett was to provide brief, structured, largely supportive group sessions to volunteer widows who had responded to newspaper descriptions of the program.

Walls and Meyers (1985) also studied three different types of time-limited, short-term group interventions. Each consisted of ten once-weekly, 90-minute sessions. One of the types was again a self-help support group that allowed members to share problems and methods of coping with the stresses of widowhood. The other two types, however, utilized techniques that have more often been used with depressed patients. The "cognitive restructuring" group focused on the negative influence of irrational thoughts and the benefits of adaptive self-verbalizations. Specific issues concerned fear of failure, social anxiety, negativism, and hopelessness about the future. The "behavioral skills" group attempted to increase the frequency and enjoyment of pleasant activities in the participants' lives. Assertiveness and social skills training were used in the groups. As did Barrett, Walls and Meyers recruited their participants from media advertisements. The two studies were also similar in that the leaders of the groups were nonwidowed, female graduate students in clinical psychology. Both the use of professionals-in-training instead of peers as leaders, and the setting of definite time limits clearly distinguished the groups of these studies from those of the self-help organizations. Features from both general approaches were used in "mutual-help" groups that were studied by Marmar, Horowitz, Weiss, Wilner, and Kaltreider (1988). In their groups, which also followed the principles of the Widow-to-Widow Program, a time limit consisting of 12 once-weekly, 90-minute sessions was used, but here the leaders were peers, that is, nonclinician widows.

Finally, Yalom and Vinogradov (1988) reported their experience conducting bereavement "support groups" that included behavioral techniques. The eight-session groups included structured exercises such as bringing a picture of the deceased spouse, or the more cognitive exercise of anticipating regret near the termination of the group. The authors, who were professional clinicians, intended the group to focus on the difficulties of the transitional stage of the normal grief reaction. They deliberately did not choose mental health clinic patients. Rather, they aimed for a general population of bereaved spouses of cancer patients at least 5 months after the death.

As highlighted at the beginning of this section, it is clear that most group intervention methods have been forms of supportive counseling rather than therapy. This has been evident by the objectives proposed, the techniques used, and the participants included in the groups. This observation suggests that there has been genuine reluctance among clinicians to provide group therapy to the bereaved. Because the Short-Term Group Therapy Program for Loss Patients of our clinical setting (McCallum & Piper, 1988) proposes to do just that, it is important to examine the bases of such apprehension. It will be argued that therapy with the bereaved can be conducted successfully in a group if certain conditions are met. In the next chapter the conditions of patient selection and preparation will be considered. In the one following Chapter 4 the conditions of composition and technique will be presented.

CHAPTER **4**

Short-Term Loss Group Program: Patient Selection and Preparation

Patients referred to the Short-Term Loss Group Program are selected by the intake therapists of the Walk-in Clinic. Sources of referral include general practitioners, friends, private psychiatrists, and social agencies. In addition, many patients are self-referred. Upon presentation patients participate in a comprehensive intake procedure, which involves several activities and typically takes a half a day to complete. First, patients complete several forms inquiring about demographic information, family background, and their reasons for seeking the clinic's services. Next, a staff therapist conducts a psychiatric assessment interview to determine a provisional diagnostic and etiologic understanding of the presenting complaint(s), with the goal of formulating an appropriate treatment plan. The assessment findings and the proposed treatment plan are then discussed with a designated staff psychiatrist. The latter then briefly interviews the patient with the therapist in attendance, whereupon the assessment and the plan for treatment are finalized.

The loss group program is appropriate for adults experiencing a pathologic reaction to loss. Whereas the initial shock has subsided, the loss continues to significantly interfere with patients' ability to enjoy a satisfying and productive life. The grief may be absent (masked), delayed, or excessive and prolonged. The loss can refer to a spouse, partner, parent, family member, or friend and can result from a separation, divorce, death, or geographical move. Many of our patients have experienced a combination of these types of losses. They are

43

offered 12 weeks of group therapy. Sessions are conducted once a week for 90 minutes. Each group is conducted by either one staff therapist or a cotherapy team who have extensive experience with psychodynamic group therapy.

Each group is composed of seven or eight patients who are expected to attend all sessions. The theoretical orientation is psychoanalytic. Hence, the debilitating effect of the loss is hypothesized as reflecting a reintensification of unconscious conflicts. Whereas a partial resolution of these conflicts may have been previously achieved, the recent experience of loss has exacerbated longstanding difficulties. We believe that the therapy group offers loss patients the opportunity to explore and negotiate a new resolution to their conflicts. Consistent with Mann's (1973) model of time-limited individual therapy, by understanding their reaction to the loss of the group upon termination of sessions, the patients may begin to work through unresolved conflicts that are associated with their previous losses. Hence, members are encouraged to explore their conflicts regarding the loss of the significant relationship and the conscious and unconscious reasons associated with its continued interference in their lives.

Selecting patients for the program involves several clinical considerations. Primarily, the therapist must identify those patients experiencing a pathologic reaction to loss. This identification is complicated by the fact that patients rarely present for psychotherapy with a self-diagnosis of pathologic grief (Lazare, 1989). Rather, loss patients tend to complain of interpersonal problems or psychiatric symptoms without reference to their precipitants. Therefore, the clinician must consider the etiology of symptoms and complaints rather than focusing solely on their phenomenology. The clinician's task can be facilitated by his or her being familiar with factors that place individuals at risk for developing a pathologic grief reaction and the indications that such a process is occurring. Although any single risk factor, symptom, or behavior is rarely sufficient to conclude that pathologic grief is present, each one can alert the clinician to pursue the contribution of past losses to patients' presentation.

The onset and course of any symptom should be explored. It is possible that the clinician will discover that the symptom's onset coincided with a loss. Symptoms that are particularly associated with pathologic grief include depression, self-destructive impulses, panic attacks, and somatic concerns. The latter may take many forms. Patients may describe a choking sensation or complain of "physical distress under the upper half of the sternum accompanied by expressions such as 'there is something stuck inside'" (Lazare, 1989, p. 391). They may complain of physical ailments reminiscent of symptoms associated with a terminal illness. Alternatively, they may present with a phobia about illness or death. When patients are asked to associate to their symptoms or phobia, the clinician often discovers that these are related to the specific illness that took the deceased.

The depression that indicates pathologic grief is typically a chronic subclinical one that is often characterized by persistent guilt and lowered self-esteem. The skilled clinician will easily note when themes of significant loss coincide with the onset of dysthymia or other presenting complaints. However, patients may identify some relatively minor loss as having triggered their symptoms of depression. This disproportionate or exaggerated grief reaction may indicate that the "minor" event has symbolic significance for the person. For example, the transfer of a supervisor may trigger a grief reaction displaced from the past loss of a parent.

Another possible indication of pathologic grief is when patients present with an unexplainable recurring sadness. When tracing the cycle of the sadness, the clinician may note that it occurs on specific dates or at certain times of the year. Somatic complaints reminiscent of symptoms associated with the terminal illness of the deceased may similarly surface on specific dates or at particular times of the year. In some cases these dates coincide with national holidays, for example, Father's Day or Christmas. In other cases there may be a more symbolic or idiosyncratic significance to the date, for example, the anniversary of the death. Somatic concerns may develop when patients reach the same age that the deceased was at the time of death (a nemesis phenomenon). The idiosyncratic nature of the events or dates that can precipitate anniversary grief reactions complicate their identification. Triggers of grief reactions with delayed onsets can be similarly obscure. Therefore, in addition to tracing the development of patients' symptoms, an etiologic formulation requires a complete family history. However, patients seldom volunteer details of significant losses when recounting their history. To determine the extent to which past losses are contributing to patients' current problems, the clinician is advised to inquire specifically about the circumstances and details of all deaths and estrangements in patients' lives. In particular, the clinician should assess each loss with respect to the presence of risk factors associated with the development of pathologic grief.

RISK FACTORS

Based on his clinical experience with 54 bereaved patients and his review of prospective studies, Parkes (1990) concluded that:

secure people whose experiences of life has led to a reasonable trust in themselves and others will cope well with anticipated bereavements, provided they are well supported by a family who respects their need to grieve. However, multiple or unexpected and untimely losses of people on whom one depends or who depended on the survivor can overwhelm the most secure person, and lack of security and support can undermine a person's capacity to cope with all types of bereavement. (pp. 309–310)

One implication of Parkes's conclusions is that there are four types of risk factors: (1) particular features of the loss, (2) the availability of social support following the loss, (3) preexisting vulnerabilities in the bereaved, and (4) the nature of the bereaved's relationship with the deceased. These risk factors are consistent with lists compiled by other authors (e.g., Lazare, 1989; Raphael & Middleton, 1990; Zisook, 1987).

1. Particular Features of the Loss. Regarding features of the loss, it has been reported that multiple, sudden, unexpected or untimely deaths can precipitate a pathologic grief reaction (Lazare, 1989; Parkes, 1990; Raphael & Middleton, 1990). The inherent risk with the aforementioned types of losses is that, presumably, the individual has not been able to prepare for the loss. Hence the ego's capacity to cope is overwhelmed. Conversely, Zisook (1987) noted that when the death of a spouse is preceded by an illness of more than 6 months, the bereaved is in danger of pathologic grief. In this latter case, presumably, the cumulative stress of dealing with a protracted illness erodes the spouse's capacity to cope. A further complication may be the survivor's guilt over feeling somewhat relieved that his or her own ordeal is finally over.

Often, in the midst of reacting to the loss of a spouse, the survivor realizes that he or she is facing a compromised financial situation (Raphael & Middleton, 1990; Zisook, 1987). This risk factor is particularly true when the death is unexpected. Often the widow or widower is simultaneously faced with losing the deceased's income, and being unable to immediately access the deceased's savings or insurance benefits, and being required to pay ongoing living expenses as well as the unexpected funeral expenses and lawyer's fees. A further complication to this risk factor may be the survivor's rage with the deceased for leaving him or her in such dire straits.

The death of a child has been proposed as the most traumatic type of loss. Its impact is not diminished even if the offspring had reached adulthood (Zisook, 1987). The risk of this type of loss seems to be related to the survivor's perception that the natural order has been contradicted: Children should bury their parents, not vice versa. In addition, those whose children die may feel a tremendous sense of inadequacy as parents. As indicated, the risk associated with the above noted features of loss may be related to the survivor's difficulty tolerating the feelings aroused by these particular circumstances. To further complicate matters, feelings of guilt, rage, or inadequacy may interfere with the survivor's acceptance of social support following such losses.

2. *Availability of Social Support Following the Loss*. Inadequate social support following a loss represents a second type of risk factor associated with the development of pathologic grief. The inadequacy may be actual or only perceived as such (Lazare, 1989). An example of actual inadequate social support occurs with recently relocated individuals such as immigrants. There are many examples where the lack of social support is only a perception or has been self-created. The bereaved may be ashamed to acknowledge that a loss has occurred, for example, following a death through suicide, AIDS, fatal accident involving a family member, or the death of an illicit lover. In some cases the bereaved may preempt the opportunity for support by invalidating the appropriateness of his or her grief, for example, following an abortion, miscarriage, or death of an ex-in-law. In other cases the loss may be even more ambiguous, for example, military personnel missing in action, the kidnapping victim, the terminally ill, or the institutionalized individual.

Perhaps the most common example of an ambiguous loss where the procurement of support is not attempted is divorce. Loss from divorce is ambiguous in that it often has occurred over a long time, making it difficult to specify what was lost and when. Because the ex-spouse is still alive, the divorced patient may invalidate his or her sense of grief. Because the divorce was pursued or accepted, the divorced patient often feels foolish acknowledging fondness for the ex-spouse and sadness over the loss.

Another type of self-imposed isolation is characterized by "the strong one" (Lazare, 1989). This type of individual typically offers support to similarly bereaved relatives and friends but cannot receive support in return. This example is similar to those who are at risk owing to their tendency to somatize under stress or to be emotionally constricted. The risk relates to their inability to effectively procure the needed support to cope with loss. When the unavailability of social support is a perception rather than a reality, the risk factor may be associated with a premorbid personality disorder.

3. *Preexisting Vulnerabilities in the Bereaved*. Personality has been hypothesized as being a key determinant of bereavement pathology

(Raphael & Middleton, 1990). It is associated with our third type of risk factor: prebereavement vulnerabilities. Most authors agree that pre-bereavement difficulties predispose an individual to further difficul-ties following loss. Those difficulties can be either psychological or physical (Zisook, 1987). As such, prebereavement depression fore-shadows a recurrent depression in reaction to loss. It is also common for loss to precipitate the manifestation of pathology in vulnerable individuals who have not exhibited significant prebereavement pa-thology. Therefore the clinician is advised to explore circumstances that may indicate a preexisting vulnerability. For example, the exis-tence of a dysfunctional family background represents a high risk factor. Parkes (1990) noted that individuals who experience pathologic grief often describe parents who were anxious, conflicted, absent, or rejecting. The link between dysfunctional backgrounds and pathologic grief can readily be understood in terms of creating deficiencies in ego development. Raphael and Middleton (1990) pointed out that neurot-icism or anxious attachment may make the bereaved so fearful of separation that extreme separation reactions to loss occur. Lazare (1989) suggested that individuals with immature or inadequate ego development are at risk because they have not attained the capacity for object constancy. The lack of object constancy may explain the heightened risk among those who have lost a parent during childhood. Often, the experience of loss as an adult can reawaken feelings associ-ated with an earlier loss (Lazare, 1989). This phenomenon can occur regardless of the significance of the current loss. Thus the person's reaction may appear somewhat exaggerated and puzzling to him or her. With careful exploration, the clinician often uncovers the symbolic connection between the past and current losses.

    4. *Nature of the Bereaved's Relationship with the Deceased.* The link between dysfunctional backgrounds and pathologic grief can also be understood in terms of object relations. When the individual's forma-tive relationships are dysfunctional or characterized by loss, he or she will reenact this type of relationship throughout life. A relationship characterized as highly ambivalent, dependent, or conflictual portends the intolerance of loss. This latter risk factor has been well documented in the clinical literature (Lazare, 1989; Parkes, 1990; Raphael & Middle-ton, 1990; Zisook, 1987). It is also well represented in theoretical writ-ings (see Chapter 2). In brief, these types of relationships reflect limited differentiation between the self and other. The loss of such a relationship is experienced, therefore, as a narcissistic injury and forebodes patho-logic grief. When assessing the type of relationship the bereaved had with the deceased, the clinician is advised to specifically explore the deceased's tendency toward alcohol and drug abuse, physical or psy-

chological abuse, gambling, and the incidence of separations and affairs. These tendencies have been associated with dependent, ambivalent, and conflictual relationships. It is important to remember that although an individual may "test positive" on one or more risk factors, the clinical manifestation of pathologic grief must be present before the grief can be designated as pathologic. To the perceptive clinician, these clues will be in evidence throughout the interview.

INDICATIONS OF PATHOLOGIC GRIEF

A pathologic grief reaction is clearly indicated when patients cannot speak of the deceased without experiencing intense and immediate grief, even though many years have passed since the loss (Worden, 1982). The grief may be characterized as excessive anger, guilt and self-blame, or depression (Parkes, 1972). Lazare (1989) concurs, noting that patients experiencing pathologic grief are often unable to discuss the deceased without crying or having their voice crack. To them it is as if the death occurred the day before, rather than months or years ago. Osterweis et al. (1984) suggested that in addition to maintaining the intensity of feeling, pathologic grief is indicated by the "active resistance to changing the feeling. Not only is there no movement but there also is a sense that the person will not permit any movement" (p. 54).

Conversely, the presence of a pathologic grief reaction may be indicated by the absence of distress following a death, despite the apparent importance of the relationship with the deceased. Indeed survivors may describe with pride how they carried on as though nothing had happened: They were busy and efficient, and may have appeared to be coping splendidly (Bowlby, 1980). Parkes (1972) suggested that this apparent absence of grief may reflect an attempt to fend off threatening emotions that are too painful to bear, for example, guilt over previous death wishes or a perceived inadequacy in loving and caring for the deceased. Hence, rather than the affect being absent, it is masked. Therefore the clinician should be alert to changes in patients' behavior at this point in the interview. They may become tense and short-tempered, responding curtly, volunteering no references to the loss. When their resistance is further explored, they often acknowledge that they have avoided reminders of the event by similarly avoiding or even forbidding references to the death within their family or social network. In this respect, to maintain the denial of the loss, patients may need to make radical changes in life-style following a death, for example, avoiding longtime friends, family, and activities associated with the deceased.

Changes occurring following a death can include taking on characteristics of the deceased, as if to imitate him or her. For example, the bereaved may become involved in a sport or activity in which the lost one engaged, despite the bereft's lack of desire or competence for the newfound interest. Worden (1982) interpreted this phenomenon as patients' attempt to compensate for the loss by identifying with the departed. Patients may begin traveling or moving from domicile to domicile and from city to city. Lazare (1989) interpreted this behavior as "searching" for the deceased. Conversely, others may wait for their return. Patients may refuse to change anything associated with the deceased. In effect they attempt to deny the loss by preserving the environment as if expecting his or her return. Horowitz (1990) has noted that the denial can continue for weeks or months following the death. We have noted that the denial can extend for years in the form of "grottoes" commemorating the deceased that exist in the homes of many patients suffering a pathologic reaction to loss.

By including in the assessment procedure an exploration of risk factors and indications of pathologic grief, the clinician can ascertain whether the patient's difficulties reflect a complicated grief reaction. This next section presents two case illustrations of representative patients selected for a group. One successfully completed the group; the other did not.

ELLEN: A SELECTION FAILURE

Ellen was a 42-year-old married housewife with three daughters. She was referred to the clinic by her general practitioner, who had been treating her with an anxiolytic medication for panic attacks for 10 months. Initially the panic disorder was experienced as a fear of going out of the house, palpitations, cold and hot flushes, tightness in the chest, and difficulty breathing. At intake she reported having resumed her usual activities, but was still experiencing palpitations. She explained her panic as a fear that her oldest child would be assaulted or kidnapped since going away to university a year ago. However, the panic had begun 2 months after the departure of her daughter, and there were no reports of dangerous incidents involving her daughter. The intake therapist explored other life circumstances that coincided with the onset of the panic. When her daughter left, a widowed aunt had moved in. They had been very close when Ellen was younger. In fact Ellen had lived with her for about 5 years before being married. When asked if they still were close, Ellen finally acknowledged, through tears, that her aunt had died 10 months ago. Ellen had invited her aunt to move in with her to nurse her through the final stages of cancer.

The intake therapist inquired about the funeral. Her daughter had not returned for it. Because the university she attended was in eastern Canada, the plane fare was considered too expensive. Her husband had made a special trip home for the funeral and Ellen was grateful for that. Her husband, Tom, was an electrician who had worked out of town for 10 years. He usually came home only on weekends. She felt that he had been supportive around the time of the funeral. Ellen and Tom's marriage 18 years ago had been precipitated by an unplanned pregnancy. Ellen stated that she liked being a housewife and enjoyed her two [sic] daughters. She denied problems associated with bringing them up virtually alone but acknowledged wishing that Tom could spend more time at home. She felt that her marriage relationship was close, with no problems. She coped with her loneliness by attending social activities. Her aunt had often accompanied her to these events.

The assessment of Ellen's family background began with questions about the circumstances under which she had gone to live with her aunt at age 19. Her family history was revealed in the same halting manner that had characterized her history of the panic disorder. Ellen was third in a sib-line of seven, with the births spanning 13 years. When Ellen was fifteen, her mother was diagnosed with cancer and became very ill. Ellen abandoned her studies in the middle of grade 9 to stay home and take care of the house, her sick mother, and her younger siblings. Two years later her mother succumbed to the cancer. Within 2 years of her mother's death, her father also died of cancer. At that point, her siblings went into separate domiciles. Ellen went to live with her aunt, who had recently lost her husband, also to cancer. Ellen worked outside the house while living with her aunt. At age 24, she became pregnant, married, and became a housewife.

In the interview Ellen denied any resentment about being deprived of an education. She explained that because she was the oldest daughter it had made sense for her to fulfill her mother's role. Concerning the death of her parents, she claimed that she had felt rather numb at the time. She explained that she was busy arranging the funeral and deciding where her sisters and brothers were going to live. When the intake therapist noted that she had in effect lost her entire family when her parents died, Ellen disagreed, stating that they had remained emotionally close despite the physical separation.

Ellen believed that the onset of her panic coincided with the departure of her daughter for university. However, the intake therapist traced her difficulties to the aunt's death. Supporting the hypothesis that pathologic grief was occurring, Ellen began to weep uncontrollably as if experiencing fresh grief when she discussed her aunt's death. In contrast, she remained calm when discussing the deaths of her parents and the departure of her daughter. The debilitating effect of the aunt's death seems to be related to several of the previously reviewed risk factors. As to the first type, particular features of the loss, there were multiple losses. The aunt died only 2 months after the daughter's departure. In addition, her death was preceded by 2 months wherein Ellen nursed her through the pain of cancer. As to the second type of risk factor, the availability of social support following the loss, there was indeed limited social support following her death. Her husband worked out of town and her daughter remained in eastern Canada. In addition, the death of her aunt represented the loss of her social companion and surrogate—probably idealized—parent. As to the third type of risk factor, preexisting vulnerabilities in the bereaved, the death of her parents represented a significant pre-bereavement vulnerability. It is hypothesized that the aunt's death exacerbated a chronic pathologic grief over the death of her parents.

Several risk factors were associated with the parents' deaths. First, regarding particular features of the loss, there were multiple losses: The father died only 2 years after the mother's death. With the parents gone, Ellen's siblings departed to different domiciles. Their departure, a loss in and of itself, also deprived Ellen of their social support. Because the aunt was recently widowed, it is doubtful that she could have offered Ellen much support at that time. Hence there was the second risk factor: inadequate social support following the deaths.

As to the third type of risk factor, preexisting vulnerabilities in the bereaved, there was evidence to suggest that Ellen was indeed a vulnerable individual. Her mother had seven children in 13 years. It is doubtful that sufficient attention was paid to all seven children. It is possible, therefore, that Ellen experienced her parents as emotionally absent. In addition, her mother's illness necessitated Ellen's with-drawal from school. She was deprived of an education and also of her youth. She was responsible for managing the household tasks and was a surrogate mother to her siblings. As reviewed in Chapter 2, Bowlby has pointed out the inhibiting effects of such a contingency on the ability to grieve normally.

An important aspect of her vulnerability concerned her personal-ity. Ellen became "the strong one." She nursed her mother before her death, she continued to care for her siblings following her death, nursed her father before his death, organized the funeral arrangements of her father, and organized the dispersion of her siblings. In effect, there was collusion by everyone to prohibit her from having the opportunity to grieve, given that she occupied herself with everyone else's welfare. There was also the suggestion of an emotional constrictiveness. She denied any resentment regarding her withdrawal from school. Rather, she rationalized, stating that "it made sense." She reported feeling "numb" after the deaths. One wonders whether the numbness masked her guilt over feeling somewhat relieved that her ordeal was over. She also denied feeling the loss of her siblings after the dispersion. Despite the lack of physical contact, she insisted that they remained emotionally close. Her reaction was somewhat consistent with the ambiguity of the loss of her siblings; they were alive but not available to her. More notably, her reaction was consistent with her tendency to deny any negative feelings. This denial precluded the procurement of support.

Ellen coped with early deprivation by developing an interpersonal stance of self-sufficiency. She continued this stance in adult life even though it meant that she continued to deprive herself of emotional support. Hence she felt obliged to nurse her aunt through the final stage of her cancer. She did not complain that she raised her daughters virtually alone. Instead she felt grateful that her husband was able to return, however briefly, for the funeral of her aunt. It is probable that by choosing a husband who was physically absent most of the time, she was able to avoid intimacy and thereby reenact her primary relationship with her parents. Furthermore, by giving her husband her blessing to remain away, she was transforming passivity into activity, albeit maladaptively.

As to the fourth type of risk factor, the nature of the bereaved's relationship with the deceased, Ellen did not describe her relationship with her parents as conflictual, dependent, or ambivalent. Given that she sacrificed her emotions, her education, and her youth for her parents, her ambivalence was conspicuously absent. Perhaps her difficulty acknowledging her ambivalence was the primary risk factor that predisposed her to pathologic grief. Her difficulty was consistent with her difficulty tolerating any emotion. By being unable to verbalize her distress, she was unable to procure support. Furthermore, she had difficulty acknowledging that she had experienced a loss. Instead she focused on the fear of losing her daughter. It is interesting that she made a slip in the interview, stating that she enjoyed her "two" daughters, as if the third were already lost by going away to university.

The intake therapist believed that the death of the aunt triggered the grief reaction displaced from her parents, especially from her mother. The trigger related to the similarities among the deaths. The aunt had been a mother figure for Ellen between the ages of 19 and 24. All three had died of cancer. Ellen had nursed all of them before their death. Finally, Ellen had denied her need to grieve in all three situations. She agreed that perhaps it was time to mourn their loss and was referred to the loss group program.

Ellen attended only one group session. Throughout that session she sat silently crying. She was unable to verbalize the strong emotions she was obviously feeling. Shaking her head silently, she discouraged attempts to include her in the group's discussion. She did not return to the group. On her own volition, she was reassessed by her intake therapist 2 months later. She denied any symptomatology or concerns. The therapist's impression was that she wanted to reassure the therapist that she was functioning very well. It is possible that Ellen's response to the experience of therapy represented a flight into health. The pain associated with beginning to experience the warded-off ideas and affects associated with her multiple losses outweighed her desire to receive help or effect change. Hence she denied the need for therapy and the difficulties that had originally brought her into treatment. It is not uncommon for patients who have terminated therapy prematurely to return later, perhaps after yet another loss, and then adhere to the original treatment plan.

MARGARET: A SELECTION SUCCESS

The second case illustration is of Margaret, a twice-divorced, currently married, 53-year-old woman working full time as an administrator. She was referred to the walk-in clinic by her family doctor, who had begun treating her with a tricyclic antidepressant one week before. She presented at the clinic complaining of "stress at work," which she attributed to friction with a new supervisor. She reported feeling "burned out" for a few months, experiencing difficulties with memory and concentration, impaired sleep, and increased tearfulness. She had difficulty describing exactly what it was about her new supervisor that she disliked. She explained that he was "just so different" from her former supervisor, who had been very warm and supportive of her. He had died suddenly 9 months earlier without her having had the opportunity to say goodbye to him.

Margaret spontaneously recounted the following history. She was the youngest of a sib-line of four. Her father had been institutionalized, apparently for bipolar disorder, when she was 2 years old. He died when she was 9 years old. She remembered no details about his death. However, both of her earliest memories involved him. The first was of him giving her his cheek to kiss. The second was of the only time he spoke to her. She does not remember what he said. The family used to visit him in the institution. She did not realize that it was a psychiatric hospital until after he died. Her mother had apparently pretended that the visits were a kind of picnic. Her mother was described as an emotionally constricted woman. Margaret emphasized that her mother had had many abortions before she was born, adding that "it doesn't make sense that she'd be happy to have me." Her mother died from Alzheimer's disease when Margaret was 40.

Margaret married three times. She met her first husband at age 16. He was 7 years her senior. They started living together almost immediately and married when she was 18, precipitated by an unplanned pregnancy. She discovered that he had had a child with his first wife. Margaret never forgave his deception and started having affairs herself. They divorced 4 years later.

At age 25, she married for a second time. That marriage was again precipitated by an unplanned pregnancy and lasted for 12 years. She described her second husband as an alcoholic who had many affairs. It was with this man that she experienced the death of four children at or around birth, owing to various birth defects. The deaths occurred within a 5-year period. After the first two deaths, Margaret delivered a healthy baby. She stated that she then became "obsessed," however, with having another baby. Six months after two more stillbirths, she successfully adopted a child. After 7 years of marriage, and with three children at home, her husband left her to return to his former wife, apparently because he missed his children from that marriage. He quickly changed his mind, however, and Margaret accepted him back. After his return, she adopted another child. Finally, his drinking and affairs eroded the relationship, and after 5 years she asked him to leave.

At age 40, Margaret started dating a married man who was 16 years her senior. He soon left his wife and married her. They have been together for 13 years. She described their relationship as "good friends." He was 69 at the time of intake and described as rather unmotivated to participate in many activities, preferring to keep to himself.

The intake therapist explored with Margaret the significance of her former supervisor. Margaret began to weep profoundly. She expressed surprise over her tearfulness, stating that she usually "coped very well" with loss. She explained the apparent lack of impact of the series of losses she had experienced in the following way: Because she hardly knew her father, she never considered his death a loss. With respect to her children, she had "kept on going" by adopting two children following the fourth stillbirth. She felt her mother's death was really a blessing and that she was well rid of her ex-husbands.

Margaret had come to the clinic believing that she was overly stressed because of friction with her new supervisor. Her "stress" was

diagnosed as clinical depression. Etiologically, there was the predisposing biological factor of her father's bipolar illness. Temporally, her
depression was related to the death of her former supervisor. The
intake therapist postulated that the depression signified a pathologic
grief reaction to the death of the supervisor. Supporting this postula-
tion, Margaret had wept uncontrollably when discussing the supervisor. It was hypothesized that the supervisor's death exacerbated a
chronic pathologic grief in reaction to her previous losses, particularly
that of her father. Her choice of husbands seemed to reflect Margaret's
hunger and search for a father. All three husbands were older and
attached to other women. The supervisor was experienced as a benev-
olent father figure. His death seemed to signify the repeated loss of
father, triggering the grief reaction.

The major risk factor associated with the death of this surrogate
father relates to prebereavement vulnerabilities. Margaret's mother was
described as an emotionally constricted woman who coped with the
loss of her husband by denying its impact. She pretended the visits were
like going on picnics. We can imagine that for a child to experience her
father as a mute, unresponsive man in a psychiatric institution would
be rather traumatic. Like her mother, Margaret disavowed her feelings
of loss regarding her father by rationalizing that she hardly knew him.
Regarding the stillbirths, she avoided her grief by quickly replacing
them with adopted children. It is possible that, given the ambiguous
nature of this latter type of loss, she may not have received adequate
social support following the deaths. The alcoholism, infidelity, and
subsequent departure of her second husband also suggest inadequate
social support at that time. Moreover, her tendency to "cope very well"
with loss probably precluded the procurement of support, because no
one would know she was in need. Hence the second type of risk factor
may have contributed to Margaret's development of pathologic grief.
Regarding the loss of her mother, she again denied any feeling except
relief. It is perhaps significant that her mother's death coincided with
her becoming involved with her third husband. It is possible, therefore,
that the loss of mother was replaced by this man. In summary, Margaret
had experienced numerous losses throughout her life. Their impact was
disavowed and they were never mourned.

Margaret's tendency to disavow her feelings of grief continued
with the loss of the supervisor. Consciously, she had focused on the
new supervisor rather than the former one. She was similarly unaware
of any ambivalence regarding any lost relationship. Her attitude was
one-sided and seemingly devoid of conflict. Her emotional reaction to
her mother's death and to her divorces was solely relief. One can
imagine that the death of her father rendered her feeling somewhat

relieved since she no longer had to partake in the picnic charades. In addition, given that her children died of profound birth defects, there may have been relief associated with nature's euthanasia. In contrast, the death of the supervisor had triggered profound sadness over this defensively idealized man. Margaret was offered a referral to a loss group. Agreeing that she had some unfinished business with the losses in her life, she accepted the referral.

Margaret attended 11 of the 12 group sessions. She ceased her medication within the first month of therapy because she associated it with "mental illness." She was a valuable group member, and in therapy she was able to express rage and sadness over the stillbirths. She also related these losses to her need for control, her anger at bosses, and her fear of intimacy. Margaret greatly benefited from the group experience. When interviewed at the end of treatment, she reported "extreme improvement" in many of the goals for which she had sought therapy. Specifically, her depression had remitted, she was no longer haunted by past losses, she was no longer overworking, and she had begun a fitness regime. Her sole complaint concerned her struggle with assertiveness in her personal relationships. When interviewed 6 months later, she reported that she had maintained the majority of the gains she had made and felt that she was being more assertive with her husband and children. Her sole complaint was that she had abandoned her fitness regime.

The puzzle for the clinician is to determine why the experiences of Ellen and Margaret were so different in the group. In terms of the patient selection criterion of pathologic grief, both were indeed exhibiting problems in reaction to unresolved past losses. It is also important to note the similarities in their backgrounds, which were rather chaotic. This chaos was typical of the loss group population and is, as mentioned, postulated as representing a predisposing and perpetuating risk factor for the development of pathologic grief. The difference between the experiences of the two women in the group seemed to be related to other criteria of suitability for the group. Those criteria are considered in the next section.

SUITABILITY CRITERIA

Woods and Melnick (1979) identified the following characteristics as inclusion criteria for group therapy: a minimum of interpersonal skill, a reasonable degree of motivation, current psychological discomfort, and reasonable expectations of gain from therapy. In terms of suitability for short-term group therapy, Poey (1985) outlined common guidelines espoused in the literature: an ability to verbalize a focal complaint, a significant level of psychological mindedness, an urge to grow and explore, a desire to enter a short-term group, realistic expectations of the group, and a basic ability to relate to and be influenced by others. Additional criteria could easily be added, such as a history of previous successful work in a group and an ability to tolerate anxiety in group situations. Criteria that have been emphasized by practitioners of dynamically oriented short-term individual psychotherapy are also relevant. Sifneos (1981) recommended that a patient possess a circumscribed chief complaint, a history of meaningful give-and-take relationships, flexible interaction with the evaluating interviewer, and above-average psychological sophistication and intelligence. These criteria are, of course, ideals. Strict adherence to all of them would preclude most patients. While general criteria such as these reflect clinical experience, it must be acknowledged that the research evidence for their validation is very limited.

Rather than assuming that general selection criteria must be made progressively restrictive as one moves from long-term to short-term forms of therapy, we believed that the nature of the patients' problems would compensate for certain "weaknesses" in general criteria. In other words, we believed that the problem of pathologic grief was particularly conducive to work and resolution in brief, time-limited group therapy. Our emphasis on this selection criterion attempted to match a patient population with a treatment form. However, our emphasis does not deny the importance of the general criteria that have been cited in the literature. After the clinician has determined that a patient is experiencing a pathologic grief reaction, other considerations for suitability are considered.

The Time-Limited Group Format

A second consideration for patient suitability for loss group is the time-limited group format. The Short-Term Group Therapy Program is not presented as a cure-all but as a therapy especially designed to focus on the issue of loss. The clinician emphasizes the support that is available from being with other people who have experienced similar losses. Suitable patients must agree to the 12 session contract and prearranged group therapy times.

The Psychoanalytic Approach

A third consideration for referral to a loss group is the psychoanalytic approach. Suitable candidates must exhibit a certain minimal level of ability and motivation to work within this approach. By interpreting the link between the presenting complaint and loss, the clinician can assess the patient's receptivity to working within this approach. Receptivity can be facilitated by pointing out the emotional evidence (e.g., tears, anger) that has surfaced throughout the interview. Suitable patients must at least agree that they have unresolved issues regarding the loss and agree to explore its impact in therapy.

Ellen and Margaret

Ellen and Margaret met the second and third clinical criteria for inclusion in the loss groups. Both agreed to attend the group and discuss their loss issues. Both appeared to the intake therapist as receptive to the psychoanalytic approach. For example, Ellen had agreed with the therapist's hypothesis that her depression was linked to her difficulty mourning the loss of her aunt. She had then explored her relationship with her aunt: the happy times; the sad times. She had smiled and wept, appropriate to the content of her recollections. Similarly, Margaret had responded to the therapist's interpretation that the loss of her supervisor was triggering feelings regarding the loss of her father. Whereas both patients were initially surprised with these dynamic formulations of their problems, they spontaneously exhibited a willingness to explore the significance of these interpretations in an emotionally meaningful way. Hence they both seemed receptive to psychoanalytic interpretations and were predicted to do well in the groups.

However, we have developed a research instrument that more deftly assesses the degree to which a patient is receptive to the psychoanalytic technique. This instrument is called the Psychological Mindedness Assessment Procedure (PMAP). The PMAP was able to discern significant differences between Ellen and Margaret in terms of their receptivity for the psychoanalytic technique. In Chapter 9 the PMAP is described and its utility for patient selection is elaborated. The differences between Ellen and Margaret discerned by the PMAP are also presented in Chapter 9.

GROUP PREPARATION

When determining that a patient is suitable for referral to loss group, the assessment process becomes interwoven with preparing the patient for the group. Careful preparation of patients is generally regarded by clinicians as an important procedure. Nevertheless, most descriptions of preparation for group therapy in the literature reveal brief, one-shot procedures. Research indicates that more elaborate procedures can improve attendance, remaining in therapy, and, possibly, the therapy process (Budman, Clifford, Bader, & Bader, 1981; Piper, Debbane, Bienvenu, & Garant, 1982; Piper & Perrault, 1989). Thus the notion that brief therapy requires only brief preparation is likely false.

Goldberg, Schuyler, Bransfield, and Savino (1983) advocated that the therapist prepare the patients individually. This method of preparation also provides the therapist with an opportunity to assess and become acquainted with the patients. A disadvantage involves the patients' reaction to the inevitable shift in the therapist's role (directive to interpretive, individual-centered to group-centered) as they proceed from preparation to therapy. Budman et al. (1981) advocated a 3-hour group preparation workshop. Although this method provides an opportunity for an assessment of the patients' capability of working in a group, it also shares the disadvantage of requiring the patients and therapist to make a considerable transition from a preparation group to a psychoanalytically oriented therapy group. In short-term groups a preparatory experience of 3 hours may be equivalent in length to nearly a quarter of the therapy group's time. In long-term groups there is considerably less need to make this transition quickly.

In the loss group program, patients receive preparation by more than one person (referring source, program interviewer) and more than one form (verbal, written). Given the emotional state of most patients anticipating group therapy, repetitive and varied preparation is much more likely to have an impact. Preparation involves discussing with the patients the group's ground rules. They include the importance of commitment and confidentiality, and suggestions as to how to comport oneself in the group (e.g., to be as honest as possible concerning thoughts and feelings experienced in the group). The form summarizing these rules are given to the patient. It is reproduced in Table 4.1.

A discussion of the ground rules offers the patient an intellectual understanding of what to expect in group. We have also experimented with a combination screening-preparation interview for three to five patients at a time. That interview is conducted by the group therapist. The advantage of this method is the similarity between preparation procedure and group experience. Patients gain an experiential understanding of what to expect in group. Similarly, the therapist may only realize that a patient is ill suited to the group after observing him or her in the group situation. As previously mentioned, the disadvantage of this method of preparation is the blurred distinction between preparation and therapy. Patients may have difficulty limiting their self-disclosures during the preparation session. Subgrouping may be indirectly encouraged by dividing the group into two separate preparation

TABLE 4.1. Ground Rules for Participation in Short-Term Group Therapy

---

Commitment:

I understand that my commitment to the group is for all 12 sessions. The group will meet for 90 minutes each week. Group attendance must be a high priority and unless there is a very good reason, such as severe illness, I will be there each week. In the event of such an absence, I will notify the therapist prior to the group and at the next meeting I will share my reason with the rest of the group. I also recognize the importance of being on time, since lateness interferes with the work of the group. If I am thinking about leaving the group, I will let others know. Should I decide to leave the group, I will come for one last session where people can say goodbye.

Responsibilities in the group:

I agree to work toward learning more about my own and others' problems. I will try to be open and self-examining. I will be as honest as possible in sharing what I am aware of in the group—that is, thoughts, feelings, fantasies—about myself, other group members (including the therapists), and other people in my life. I understand that I cannot come to group under the influence of alcohol or drugs. It is also not permissible to smoke, drink, or eat in group. I also understand that physical violence will not be tolerated in the group.

Responsibilities outside the group:

Confidentiality is essential so that each member can feel safe enough to share. I agree that I will not repeat anything that is said in the group outside of it, unless it concerns only myself. I will not share information that might identify any member of the group. Extra group socializing may prevent the work in the group. I understand that contact with another member (including the therapist) outside of group may sabotage my own treatment and I agree to discuss the details of any chance outside contacts in the group.

---

groups. Therapists may feel uncomfortable shifting from the more educational, directive stance utilized during preparation to the more psychoanalytically oriented, nondirective stance utilized during therapy. The majority of therapists at our clinic feel that the screening aspect of the preparation group compensates for their discomfort in shifting from the preparation to the therapeutic stance.

EXCLUSION CRITERIA

In practical terms, a discussion of patient selection criteria and preparation procedures involves a consideration of exclusion criteria. As with any psychodynamic group, patients who are suicidal, psychotic, severely depressed, or who have current substance abuse problems are not considered suitable. Suicidal, severely depressed, and psychotic patients may need to be hospitalized if they represent an imminent danger to themselves or others. If treated on an outpatient basis, they are offered a psychopharmacologic intervention and seen for individual, supportive sessions until they no longer constitute a danger. Whereas these sessions need only last 10 or 15 minutes each, for some patients they need to be conducted on a daily basis. For those patients with current substance abuse problems a referral to the province of Alberta Alcohol and Drug Abuse Commission is offered. After the symptoms that render these patients unsuitable have been counteracted, they can be reconsidered for group treatment.

For our psychoanalytically oriented loss groups, we normally exclude individuals who are experiencing an uncomplicated mourning process. Instead they are offered support and problem-solving strategies through individual crisis intervention sessions. They may also be referred to community agencies. For example, if the death was due to Sudden Infant Death Syndrome (SIDS), the patient is offered a referral to a SIDS support group; if the death was due to Autoimmune Deficiency Syndrome (AIDS), the patient is referred to the AIDS Network, which offers support groups for survivors. In general, therefore, for patients referred to the groups, the loss has not occurred during the past 3 months. Selecting patients for short-term group based on the identification of a pathologic grief reaction has implications for group composition and therapist technique. These are addressed in the next chapter.

CHAPTER **5**

Group Composition and Therapist Technique

$\mathbf{T}$his chapter focuses on two additional conditions that are important to the successful implementation of short-term loss groups. The first is group composition, which refers to the general makeup of the group in terms of patient characteristics. The second is therapist technique, which refers to the nature of the interventions provided by the therapist. Although it may seem that these two conditions represent very different aspects of a therapy group, it will be argued that they are inextricably related in the case of short-term loss groups. This is largely due to two factors. In the formation of loss groups, substantial effort is exerted to create homogeneous group composition, in other words, groups where many patient characteristics are shared. In turn, therapists devote considerable attention to group—that is, shared—processes through their interventions. If homogeneous composition is achieved and the patient characteristics are known, the therapist is in a good position to predict certain group processes and be ready to make appropriate interventions. Similarly, a knowledge of group composition coupled with a theoretical understanding of the patients' problem areas can enhance the therapist's sensitivity to minimal cues provided by the patient about important issues, as well as sensitivity to the absence of such cues. In the latter case the therapist can interpret the avoidance of certain topics. In short-term loss groups, group composition has a profound effect in setting the stage for therapist interventions.

GROUP COMPOSITION

Certainly more obvious than the relationship between group composition and therapist technique is the relationship between patient
selection and group composition. Patient selection directly determines
the composition of the group. Pertinent to the link between the two in
the case of dynamically oriented short-term group therapy is Goldberg, Schuyler, Bransfield, and Savino's (1983) recommendation that
"the central principle governing patient selection is broad-based homogeneity, including the establishment of a common theme" (p. 423).
Broad-based homogeneity can be defined as patient commonalities on
a number of variables. These may include personality characteristics,
presenting problems, life events, demographic characteristics, and
underlying conflicts. Goldberg et al. noted that a concerted effort to
achieve broad-based homogeneity in short-term therapy groups is a
significant modification of customary procedures, for example, those
followed in the case of dynamically oriented long-term group therapy.
The more traditional position is represented by Whitaker and Lieberman (1964), who state that "maximum heterogeneity in the patient's
position on specific conflict areas appears to be desirable" (p. 205).
Within the term *conflict area* they include both content and coping
mechanisms. In regard to homogeneity they recommend that patients
be homogeneous in vulnerability, for example, their capacity to tolerate anxiety. The degree of patient heterogeneity that can be tolerated
and used beneficially in a therapy group appears to be related to the
group's time structure. What proves to be stimulating in a long-term
therapy group may prove to be distracting in a short-term therapy
group.

   If one accepts the desirability of achieving patient homogeneity in
short-term group therapy, the practical question that arises next is
which patient characteristics should be given priority. It is assumed
that it is not possible to achieve homogeneity on all variables. One
dimension that should be considered is the level of abstractness versus
concreteness of the variables. If commonality is conceptualized at an
abstract level—for example, a certain type of unconscious conflict—
the range of suitable patients is broader. The risk with this approach is
that patients may have difficulty identifying with each other owing to
the heterogeneous manner in which the conflict manifests itself. This
may be the case despite the clarity of the conflict in the therapist's
mind. However, if commonality is conceptualized at a more concrete
level such as overt symptomatology and interpersonal difficulties, the
group process may remain at a superficial descriptive level. Interpretation and understanding may be hampered because a variety of

different conflicts may give rise to similar symptomatology and inter-personal difficulties.

A proposed solution to the problem of selecting patient character-istics for homogeneous group composition is to choose variables at more than one level of abstraction. Thus, rather than limiting the homogeneity of the group to one portion of the abstract-concrete dimension, a combination of characteristics at different levels is pref-erable. This strategy has been used with reported success by Budman, Bennett, and Wisneski (1981) in their work with short-term therapy groups in Boston. For example, in their young adult groups, patients share the concrete and obvious commonalities of age and life stage. In addition, at a more abstract level they are assumed to share central conflicts concerning intimacy versus isolation. The difficulties that they experience and discuss in their group are regarded as typical of their age and representative of their shared conflicts concerning inti-macy. The presence of both concrete and abstract commonalities al-lows the group to work with a wide range of phenomena.

In our short-term loss group program we have attempted to employ a similar strategy. Patients in the loss groups share common-alities at several levels of abstraction. At a more concrete level they share an obvious historical event, the loss of a person. Whereas the type of person that has been lost may differ (parent, child, partner), as may the circumstances of loss (death, divorce), the common event of losing someone is a great equalizer. Also, at a relatively concrete level, patients share familiar types of symptomatology and dysfunction. Loss patients typically experience sadness, anger, loneliness, low self-esteem, and a sense of social isolation. When patients speak of their feelings and experiences, others know what they mean. At a more abstract level, patients share long-standing conflicts. Those concerning dependence versus independence and intimacy versus privacy seem to be typical of loss patients. Given a definite set of commonalities at different levels of abstraction, we have found that the groups can tolerate variability on other patient demographic characteristics such as age and sex as well as type of loss—for example, death versus divorce.

The presence of commonalities at multiple levels greatly facilitates the development of "universality," that is, a sense of shared experi-ence, which is a curative factor that Yalom (1985) and others have repeatedly cited as being important to progress in group therapy. Another curative factor that no doubt is strengthened by multiple patient commonalities is cohesion. By cohesion we mean the various bonds that become established between a given patient and other patients, the therapist, and the group as a whole (Piper, Marrache,

Lacroix, Richardsen, & Jones, 1983). We have repeatedly been impressed with how quickly patients self-disclose and become affectively involved in the loss groups. In a short-term group where time is limited, this is an important benefit. A sense of trust needs to develop quickly if the challenging and, at times, anxiety-arousing aspects of psychodynamic work are to take place in the group.

THERAPIST TECHNIQUE

Patient selection, patient preparation, and group composition for short-term loss groups require a significant investment of time and clinical skill to be implemented properly. The task of leading the groups is even more demanding, however, than selecting, preparing, and composing patients for the groups. The very combination of features that make the short-term loss group program unique—psychoanalytically oriented therapy in a group setting with a short-term time limit—is what creates the primary challenge for the therapist. If the therapy were carried out without the group situation (individually), without the time limit (open-ended), or without the short-term duration (many months), pressure on the therapist would be much less. Thus, owing to the time constraints of therapy, the therapist simply cannot afford to be passive. However, maintaining an active presence, which we refer to technically as "consistent focusing," runs the risk of violating certain technical principles that are often associated with the psychoanalytic orientation. The shifting priorities involving these technical principles must be managed by the therapist throughout the life of the group. Thus the role required of the therapist is an energy-consuming one, which at times can be quite stressful. Before examining the therapist's role more closely, let us consider certain characteristics of the psychoanalytic orientation.

As a part of previous projects with colleagues in Montreal, a set of criteria for defining the term *psychoanalytic work* was published in 1986 in an article by Bienvenu, Piper, Debbane, and de Carufel. These criteria were modifications of Merton Gill's intrinsic criteria for psychoanalysis (Gill, 1954, 1984). The modifications permitted application of the criteria to different forms of psychotherapy (short-term, long-term, individual, and group). Some of the criteria focused on the patient and some on the therapist. Those that focused on the therapist included (1) passive encouragement of the regressive process of the patient, (2) maintenance of a position of neutrality, (3) analysis of transference as a central aim, and (4) use of interpretation as the main technique to resolve conflicts. The criteria that focused on the patient concerned the patient's ability and willingness to engage in the regressive process and to work with interpretation as the main technique. Taken as a whole, the criteria cover a regressive process, a technical process, and a progressive process.

The criteria as delineated by Bienvenu et al. are considered to be ideals, which, as such, are never fully achieved. The more fully they are achieved, the more that psychoanalytic work can be said to be occurring and the more a particular form of therapy can be regarded as psychoanalytic in nature. Given the demanding nature of psychoanalytic work under even the most optimal conditions, it is reasonable to wonder whether such work is possible to accomplish when the time for therapy is limited and the situation involves a group modality. In every group the demands on the participants are coupled with inevitable tensions concerning control, individuality, understanding, privacy, and safety. Under these circumstances resistance to interpretive work can be expected as a matter of course. As those authors point out, part of the task of the therapist is to constantly try to understand failures at achieving these ideals in order to provide new interpretations that can help restore a new proximity to the intrinsic criteria. This is considered to be a continuous process.

The criteria that focus on the therapist guided the technical approach used with short-term therapy groups that were part of a comparative outcome study conducted in Montreal (Piper, Debbane, Bienvenu, & Garant, 1984). Four forms of psychotherapy were studied: short-term individual, long-term individual, short-term group, and long-term group. The short-term groups met once a week for 6 months. The groups were not loss groups, however. The patients represented a more heterogeneous sample of psychiatric outpatients who suffered from neurotic or mild-to-moderate characterological problems. The therapists were three male psychiatrists who had 12, 6, and 2 years of postqualification (Fellow, Royal College of Physicians, Canada) experience treating patients with individual and group psychotherapy. All three were psychoanalytically oriented, two having received formal training from a psychoanalytic institute. Thus the therapists were an experienced team for whom the practice of outpatient therapy represented a major portion of their professional work.

In each case the therapist's technical approach to both the short-term and long-term group therapies of the project was similar. A relatively inactive therapist role was planned and carried out. Pressures to provide immediate gratification to the patients in the form of attention and praise were resisted. At times the therapist's technical approach contributed to a climate of deprivation which stimulated regressive processes. Accordingly, patient anxieties and conflicts that were related to their long-term difficulties were allowed to emerge. In the here-and-now group situation they could be examined by the participants and interpreted by the therapist. Pointing out similarities in problematic situations that involved past significant others, current significant others outside the group, as well as the members of the group, was part of the therapist's task. This required careful attention to transference phenomena. The therapists also attempted to maintain a neutral position in which self-disclosure was avoided. The overall technical approach, which reflected adherence to the criteria, was characteristic of approaches to dynamically oriented long-term group psychotherapy as it commonly has been practiced in North America. Evidence documenting the effectiveness of the approach in long-term groups from both clinical reports and research studies can be found in the literature (Piper, Debbane, & Garant, 1977).

Evidence for the effectiveness of the long-term groups in the Montreal comparative study was of two types. One type involved the therapists' impression of the therapy process, which was clearly positive. As the therapists reported, therapy was characterized by a high degree of involvement and attentiveness by both patients and therapists. The presence of a group of people provided continual stimulation. There was ample time to deal with important issues that were not immediately and directly associated with the patient's presenting symptomatology. Overall, the clinical material was regarded as rich and varied. The active involvement and attentiveness for both patients and therapists seemed to have facilitated an optimal mobilization of affect on the patient's part. In addition to the impressions of the therapy process, a comprehensive battery of outcome measures was used to assess therapy outcome in the comparative project. Although there was some evidence for significant improvement associated with each of the four forms of therapy, it was also clear that the results favored long-term group therapy and short-term individual therapy over long-term individual therapy and short-term group therapy.

In general, the poorest outcome results were associated with short-term group therapy. If it had been studied alone, its results would have appeared more favorable. In relation to the other three forms of therapy, however, its results were disappointing. The therapists' impressions of the therapy process were consistent with the outcome results. Both the patients and the therapists experienced difficulties. The therapy seemed to heighten the patients' anxiety about obtaining relief for their problems to the exclusion of allowing themselves to engage in an exploration of relationship difficulties experienced in the group. Initial anxiety about working on sensitive issues in the presence of others was soon followed by anxiety about ending the group. An uncomfortable atmosphere of deprivation was predominant. The therapists felt burdened with the task of trying to treat 7–8 patients together for their presenting problems using a psychoanalytically oriented approach in the limited time and situation that was available. A sense of too little time permeated the groups; hence the levels of involvement, attentiveness and affect were far from optimal.

Although the results for the short-term groups in the comparative study were disappointing, the investigators suspected that other technical applications of psychoanalytically oriented therapy in short-term groups might prove more successful. That idea was consistent with recommendations that were being made in the literature about adapting psychoanalytically oriented therapy to a short-term group format (Goldberg et al., 1983; Poey, 1985). The recommendations included the encouragement of rapid group cohesion, the maintenance of a clear and specific focus, an emphasis on awareness of the time limit, an active therapist role, and a focus on current relationships and behavior (particularly as they occur in the group). These recommendations and our experience with the short-term groups of the Montreal comparative study were quite influential in determining the technical guidelines for short-term loss groups to be carried out in Edmonton. Clearly we did not want to repeat an approach that might lead to disappointing treatment results. At the same time we wished to maintain and test a psychoanalytic orientation.

Based on our previous experience as well as the consensus in the literature on the topic, a more active therapist role seemed highly indicated. In contrast to conducting long-term group therapy, a short-term group therapist cannot afford to accumulate substantial evidence prior to interpreting, nor can he or she afford to let the group engage in lengthy defensive maneuvers before intervening. The therapist must be ready and able to offer interpretations based upon considerable inference. This may create a dilemma for traditionally trained psychodynamic therapists who have been taught to accumulate substantial evidence before making interpretations and to avoid manipulating patients and revealing themselves. Indeed, the two psychoanalytic criteria that appear to be in the most danger of being violated by a more active therapist role are the passive encouragement of regression and the neutral position of the therapist. The more that such criteria are violated, the greater the danger that the process involves persuasion rather than psychoanalytic work.

After much consideration we came to the conclusion that the two criteria might be preserved if the therapists in their active role take as much care in what they do *not* say as in what they do say. Stated in different terms, greater activity, does not have to involve greater immediate gratification or greater self-disclosure. If the therapists are clear about what types of interventions are required and are experienced enough and well trained to use clinical material to make interventions, then lapses into immediate gratification and self-revelation might be avoided. We also believed that particular types of required interventions (e.g., interpretations about group events) might serve to preserve aspects of passive encouragement and neutrality. We were aware that the aim of preserving the criteria rested upon a number of "ifs" and "mights." Whereas success in carrying out the intended technical approach could be facilitated by employing experienced therapists who followed clear technical guidelines, such success could not be guaranteed. Convincing evidence of technical adherence requires a thorough content analysis of therapy session material. This is one of the reasons why such an analysis was conducted with a large number of the groups in the Edmonton program. It will be presented in Chapters 8 and 9.

Although passive encouragement of the regressive process and maintenance of a position of neutrality appear to be the criteria at greatest risk for violation with an active therapist role, the other two criteria, analysis of transference as a central aim and use of interpretation as the main technique, are also at risk. These technical features address sensitive material and must be provided in a manner that invites work rather than resistance. Their content needs to be based upon evidence from the group, and the timing of their delivery is important. If offered without evidence or prematurely, they will not facilitate psychoanalytic work. Because of their importance, the concepts of interpretation and transference will be reviewed prior to elaborating the overall role of the therapist in short-term loss groups.

Interpretation

In the field of psychoanalytically oriented psychotherapy, the term *interpretation* has had two related, but different, usages. The first concerns the process in the therapist's mind whereby meaning is attributed to the patient's verbal and behavioral productions. In accordance with the principle of psychic determinism, the patient is viewed as ultimately understandable even if his or her experiences and behavior may seem to defy understanding. From efforts to understand dreams, the distinction between latent (or hidden) meaning and manifest (or evident) meaning gained importance. Theoretically it was assumed that the patient was unaware of the latent meaning of dreams, fantasies, motivation, behavior, and other experiences. Because of their unacceptable aspects, internal defensive processes were assumed to disguise the latent content, and therefore, to produce the manifest content. Presumably, an objective party such as a therapist could observe the manifest content, and with the help of free association by the patient and the therapist's theoretical knowledge, skill, and experience, come to understand the latent content, that is, its meaning. Once this had been accomplished, the second usage of the term interpretation would become relevant. This refers to the communication of the latent meaning to the patient.

At first it was thought that the therapist's understanding of the latent meaning could be immediately followed by communication to the patient. With experience, however, it became evident that much more had to be considered for an interpretation to have an optimal impact. This included the affective state of the patient, ongoing defensive processes, resistance, and transference. Also, the kind of information conveyed and the order in which it is conveyed had to be considered. Thus appropriate timing came to be emphasized. These developments in technique coincided with theoretical advances in the field such as the shift from the topographic model of the mind, where the purpose of interpretation was to make the unconscious conscious, to the structural model, where the purpose was to enhance the ego's mastery of id, superego, and external reality. From the latter perspective an interpretation attempted to present what was not yet in words, but what was about or likely to become words, thereby enlarging the ego's boundaries and its mastery of what was previously unknown.

As the field developed, it became clear that interpretations could not be viewed as independent statements. The boundaries of an interpretation are often difficult to delimit. According to Rycroft (1958), every statement implies two other classes of statements: (1) the assumptions that had to be made before formulating the statement, and (2) the corollary statement that can be deduced from it. Loewenstein (1951) spoke of the necessary preparatory process that culminates in the giving of an interpretation. He mentioned preparation, confrontation, and clarification. Bibring (1954) also distinguished clarification from interpretation. Greenson (1967) differentiated between confrontation, clarification, and interpretation. Others (Freud, 1937/1964; Rosen, 1977) distinguished interpretation from construction. Although there are similarities in some of the authors' distinctions, they are far from identical. To further complicate matters, Loewenstein and others made the valid point that interpretations are often given in installments as therapy proceeds. A series of statements, each making reference to some part of a dynamic equation, (e.g., defense, anxiety, or wish), might be given before an attempt at integration is made. Even though such a progression is quite reasonable, it can make recognition of an interpretation somewhat difficult, particularly in light of the overlapping terminology in the field.

Our own efforts over a number of years to differentiate therapist interpretations from other interventions led us to develop a formal classification system. It is called the Therapist Intervention Rating System (TIRS). An article describing the system was published in the *Bulletin of the Menninger Clinic* (Piper, Debbane, de Carufel, & Bienvenu, 1987). As part of the system, we wanted to provide a definition of interpretation that was both meaningful and operational. Such a definition clearly has the potential to facilitate research about therapist interpretations, and several research applications are described in that article. Two other benefits were less obvious initially, but became apparent as time went on. The first was the degree to which our definition contributed to clearer conceptual thinking about the role of interpretation in psychoanalytic psychotherapy. This became quite important when we considered the more complex group therapy situation. The second was the degree to which our definition was useful in training therapists both to practice psychoanalytic psychotherapy and to follow the research project's technical manual. Training was an important activity at both the Montreal and Edmonton clinical settings.

Because of the centrality of the concept of conflict in psychoanalytic theory, we decided to give it particular emphasis in our definition of interpretation. To qualify as an interpretation in the TIRS, a therapist intervention had to address the notion of conflict. Conflict can be considered from one or more of the five different psychoanalytic points of view, namely, topographic, dynamic, economic, structural, and genetic (Fenichel, 1945). Although all five are applicable, certain of the points of view (topographic, dynamic) are more evident in clinical material. By requiring less abstraction they are more amenable to the formulation of a clear working definition. While a definition of interpretation based upon the topographic point of view (e.g., a statement that makes conscious what was unconscious) has a simple conceptual appeal, it is also problematic. Trying to decide whether a statement brought something into consciousness is a very difficult task. In addition, the division between the unconscious and the preconscious does not adequately reflect different aspects of the conflictual situation. An interpretation of something unconscious (descriptive unconscious) might not touch on a conflictual situation, or an interpretation might refer to certain conflictual drive derivatives that are conscious, because not all defenses operate in such a way as to bar them from consciousness. Such limitations led us to reject the topographic point of view as the basis of our definition of interpretation.

What we chose for the basis of our definition of interpretation was the dynamic point of view, which explains mental phenomena as the result of interacting forces. In actuality the dynamic point of view is frequently linked with the topographic point of view in definitions of interpretation (Laplanche & Pontalis, 1967/1973). An interpretation from the dynamic point of view can be said to express the content of what is repressed, for example, a wish giving rise to anxiety acting as a signal to mobilize defenses. In practice one could accept as a minimum definition of an interpretation a statement that reveals one or more aspects of the dynamic equation in the context of a conflictual situation. This is the position we adopted.

According to the TIRS, an intervention is defined as any statement made by the therapist. Interpretations are the subclass of interventions that refer to one or more dynamic components that are part of an internal conflict. In individual psychotherapy internal means within the patient (intrapsychic). A dynamic component is part of the patient that exerts an internal force on some other part(s) of the patient. Common examples are wish, anxiety, and defense, although any affect, behavior, or cognition of the patient can have a dynamic impact on some other part of the patient. An example of an interpretation that refers to a wish and a defense is "You want to succeed, but you end up devaluing your achievements." In individual psychotherapy, if the impact of part of the patient is only upon someone else, it is not defined as a dynamic component. In group psychotherapy the definitions are somewhat expanded. Internal means within the group instead of just within the individual. A dynamic component is part of one or more patients that is exerting an internal force on one or more patients in the group or the group as a whole. The impact can be intrapsychic or interpersonal. An example of the latter is "The women's expression of anger about what they have lost seems to have silenced the men." In group psychotherapy, if the impact of part of one or more patients is only upon someone outside the group, it is not defined as a dynamic component. In the short-term loss group program, familiarity with the TIRS has proven to be quite useful to the therapists in clarifying the distinction between interpretations and other types of interventions.

Transference

A focus on transference, like that on interpretation, has been regarded as a hallmark of psychoanalytically oriented psychotherapy.

When they occur together the therapist is said to have given a transference interpretation. A well-known general definition of transference was provided by Greenson (1967):

> Transference is the experience of feelings, drives, attitudes, fantasies, and defenses toward a person in the present which do not befit that person but are a repetition of reactions originating in regard to significant persons of early childhood, unconsciously displaced onto the figures in the present. (p. 171)

According to Greenson, the cardinal features of transference are its repetition of the past and its inappropriateness to the present.

In reviewing the concept of transference some 20 years ago, Sandler, Dare, and Holder (1970) concluded that different psychoanalytic authors advocated rather different definitions of transference. The same conclusion can be made today. At a theoretical level there is disagreement about what the concept encompasses and what additional concepts (e.g., therapeutic alliance, real relationship) are needed to account for the patient's reaction (Ehrenreich, 1989). There is also disagreement about the degree to which transference should be viewed as an enactment of an earlier relationship or a new experience (Cooper, 1987). At a technical level there are differences of opinion about the importance of including developmental (genetic) material in transference interpretations, in contrast to focusing solely on the here and now interaction. These issues are relevant to both individual and group forms of psychotherapy.

In individual psychotherapy transference concerns the patient's distorted reactions to the therapist. In group psychotherapy the concept has been broadened to include the patient's distorted reactions to other patients in the group. Some have referred to this as lateral transference. Although different theoretical and technical positions have been taken, there is general agreement that insight into the meaning of the patient's reactions to other persons is a potent therapeutic ingredient. Because the reaction occurs in the here-and-now, the extent to which it is repetitious and inappropriate can be explored in a situation that is immediate and compelling. As Yalom (1985) has stated in the case of group therapy, "What better way to help the patient recapture the past than to allow him or her to reexperience and reenact ancient feelings toward parents through the current relationship to the therapist?" (p. 200). A similar statement can be made regarding siblings and other patients in the group.

THE THERAPIST ROLE IN THE
SHORT-TERM LOSS GROUPS

In practicing psychotherapy one finds there are always differences between intentions and realizations. The degree to which our therapists actually succeeded in adhering to the technical guidelines initially established for the loss groups will be addressed in Chapter 8. There the results of a content analysis involving the 16 groups that were part of the clinical evaluation will be presented. The role of the therapist as described in the present section represents what the therapists attempted to achieve.

It was clearly the therapists' intention to provide a psychoanalytic form of psychotherapy. Therefore an attempt was made to respect the criteria for psychoanalytic therapy as delineated by Bienvenu et al. (1986). With regard to the first criterion (passive encouragement of the regressive process of the patient), the therapist was passive at the onset of each session. Responsibility for deciding how to begin the session and what to talk about was left to the patients. Given the dependent traits of many of the patients, this way of beginning each session tended to increase their anxiety levels and trigger regressive processes. As indicated earlier in this chapter, as the session progressed the therapist became quite active. Certain types of interventions, however, were deliberately avoided. The therapist continued to avoid making directives about what should be discussed in the group. Silences that occurred during the session were rarely broken by the therapist. Questions directed to the therapist were rarely responded to with a simple answer. Immediate gratification in the form of special attention, praise, or smiles was avoided. Questions directed to individual patients by the therapist were used sparingly. These technical features served to create a steady pressure on the patients of the group to provide spontaneous, here-and-now material for exploration and interpretation.

With regard to the second criterion (maintenance of a position of neutrality), the therapist attempted to avoid making judgments and personal disclosures that included historical information and affective reactions. It was not uncommon for patients to want to know whether the therapist had also suffered losses. They were not provided with such information. The high activity level of the therapist, of course, made maintenance of a position of neutrality more of a challenge than if a more passive role had been adopted.

The third and fourth criteria (analysis of transference as a central aim; use of interpretation as the main technique to resolve conflicts) address what the therapist attempted to do rather than what the therapist attempted to avoid. Interpretation was the primary activity. Analysis of transference, even when expanded to include lateral transference to other patients in the group, was for the most part a small subset of the overall interpretive activity of the therapist. The therapist would listen carefully to the free-flowing interaction in the group, attempt to make sense of it, and attempt to make an interpretation as previously defined. That is, the therapist would attempt to make a statement about one or more dynamic components that are part of a conflict at an intrapsychic or interpersonal level in the group. Whenever possible, the evidence for the interpretation was also provided.

Certain conflicts that had particular relevance to loss (dependence vs. independence, privacy vs. intimacy) were frequently targeted. In retrospect, after conducting and reviewing many of the loss groups it became apparent to us that a similar set of conflicts had emerged and had received interpretations in many of the groups. We chose the term "theme" to refer to the specific content of such conflicts that exist in a group over a period of time. We also became aware that similar patient roles had emerged in many of the groups. The term "role" referred to a well-defined set of behaviors presented by a patient that represents a conflict shared by other patients. The concepts of theme and role helped sharpen our thinking about the emergence of conflictual material in the group. They will be dealt with in more detail, including specific examples, in Chapter 6. As to therapist technique, we believe that familiarity with recurrent themes and roles enhances the early recognition of their presence in the group and the provision of relevant interpretations. Given the time constraints associated with loss groups, a well-primed therapist is likely to be a more skillful one.

In addition to the four psychoanalytic criteria so far considered, two other technical criteria have guided the therapists. They were important because of the particular features that characterized the short-term loss groups. These features were the homogeneous group situation, the short-term time limit, and the topic of loss. We have labeled the two criteria "consistent focus upon commonalities" and "use of structural limitations."

The term *commonalities* refers to characteristics that patients share. Obvious examples are those features that were used to achieve homogeneous composition, that is, the historical event of person loss, symptomatology and dysfunction, and long-standing conflicts. In addition, there are the multitude of events and experiences that occur in the therapy group itself. In general the therapist used commonalities to address more than one patient or the group-as-a-whole rather than only one patient. In this way the therapist attempted, effectively as well as affectively, to involve most if not all of the patients through each "group" interpretation. The group situation permitted this particular technical emphasis.

With regard to the second of the additional criteria, limited time and the group situation are definite structural limitations of the short-term loss groups. A question of importance is whether by the use of appropriate technique they can be transformed into assets. The time limit of the group is a particularly relevant issue for loss patients. They join the group knowing that they will lose the group and the relationships therein after a brief period of time. Proponents of time-limited therapy have argued that "existential" concerns about limitations accelerate therapeutic processes. Certainly termination of the group represents an opportunity for patients to examine their own and others' reactions to an immediate loss and to compare them with previous reactions, which often have been conflictual and unresolved. In addition, more adaptive responses can be attempted. For these reasons the therapist attempted to continue to highlight the time limit and the issues associated with it. This occurred at the beginning of the group as well as at the end, where it received particular emphasis.

The group situation provides less individual attention to patients than in the case of individual psychotherapy. This limitation creates tensions concerning neglect and abandonment by authority figures and questions concerning the value that should be attributed to peer assistance. Many loss patients have manifested dependent traits, if not personality disorders, and have sought ready substitutes for the people they have lost. Dependent expectations regarding the therapist and frustration about his or her behavior are typical patient responses. Other limitations associated with the group situation include absenteeism and dropping out by some group members. Such events trigger feelings and conflicts that are similar to the reactions that patients experienced toward persons they feared losing, were losing, or in fact had lost. Accordingly, the therapist attempted to highlight these limitations associated with the group situation. We believe that unless the concerns associated with the structural limitations of short-term loss groups are directly addressed, and when possible linked to the presenting problems of patients, the limitations will function more as liabilities than assets.

In summary, the role required of the therapist in short-term loss groups is a demanding one. The therapist must maintain an active presence largely through interpretive rather than supportive techniques. Repeatedly confronting patients with conflictual material often engenders resistance. At times it may seem as if some patients have not understood or even heard what was offered. Passively encouraging regressive processes, maintaining a position of neutrality, highlighting transference phenomena, and addressing the group rather than individuals certainly does not make one immediately popular with patients. Direct expressions of appreciation for one's role are infrequent even at the end of the group. The same time pressure that patients experience is felt by the therapist. As indicated earlier, the role required of the therapist is an energy-consuming one that at times can be quite stressful. Counterbalancing these difficult aspects of the therapist role are several factors. The first is the subjective impression when conducting loss groups that the technical features and structure of the loss groups seem to fit the patients and the type of problems that they present. The second is the conceptual rationale for the technical features, which is logically consistent with the aim of addressing problems related to loss. The third and probably most important factor is the evidence that supports the effectiveness of the groups. The evidence from the formal research evaluation will be presented in Chapter 8. Prior to that, however, we will consider a clinical illustration of one of the loss groups (Chapter 6) and will review the evidence concerning the effectiveness of other group intervention methods with persons suffering from loss (Chapter 7).

CHAPTER **6**

A Clinical Illustration of a Short-Term Therapy Group for Loss

Different stages of short-term groups have been espoused in the literature (Goldberg, Schuyler, Bransfield, & Savino, 1983; MacKenzie & Livesley, 1983). For example, in his recent book on time-limited group psychotherapy MacKenzie (1990) identified six major stages: engagement, differentiation, individuation, intimacy, mutuality, and termination. Each is associated with different tasks. Others have identified an even greater number of stages, for example, Beck (1974) differentiated nine. Despite differences in the number of stages described, there is considerable agreement among the investigators as to the general nature of the stages. Those investigators who describe a greater number of stages tend to further subdivide some of the stages of those who describe a fewer number.

In the short-term loss groups we have found it useful to distinguish three major stages: the beginning, sessions one through three; the middle, sessions four through eight; and the termination, sessions nine through twelve. It should be understood that this grouping of sessions into stages is intended as an approximation, in that each group proceeds at its own pace. Each stage can be seen as presenting the group with particular tasks and obstacles that require different strategies and responses for goal attainment. In this chapter we offer a clinical illustration of one of the psychoanalytically oriented short-term loss groups (STG) from our program as it evolved through the beginning, middle, and termination stages. We present three vignettes that correspond to the three stages of group development. The vignettes include transcriptions of the patients' statements as well as the therapist's interventions.

These three clinical vignettes reflect common themes that we have found to emerge in each STG we have conducted. By "theme" we refer to the specific content of a conflict that exists in the group over a period of time. Our definition is more inclusive than that of Whitaker and Lieberman (1964) because it refers to all components of a conflict, not just the wish. We have noted characteristic themes that recur throughout the life of the group and other themes whose emergence seem to be associated with specific events or stages of the group. Both types of group themes are represented by the clinical material to follow.

The first vignette depicts the beginning stage of a group, and our discussion of this material focuses on the therapist's role and activity. The second depicts the middle stage of the same group, and our discussion of this material focuses on characteristic patient behavior. The third depicts the group's termination stage, and our discussion of this material focuses on themes associated with termination.

THE GROUP

The group that is presented in this chapter consisted of seven patients and one female therapist. There were five women and two men in the group. Two of the group members, Margaret and Ellen, have been described in detail in Chapter 4. A brief description of those members will be repeated here to refresh the reader's memory.

Margaret: This 53-year-old administrator presented at the clinic complaining of "stress of work" attributed to friction with a new supervisor. Her former supervisor had died suddenly 9 months before. Margaret's history revealed that she had "coped very well" with the death of her father when she was 9 years old, the loss of four children at or around birth owing to various birth defects, and her two divorces.

Ellen: This member was a 42-year-old married housewife with three children. She presented at the clinic complaining of panic attacks following the death of her aunt 10 months before. Ellen's history revealed that her mother had died when she was 17 years old and her father had died when she was 19.

The other five members consisted of:

Alice: The third member was a 29-year-old receptionist. She complained of chronic low self-esteem, which she attributed to leaving school at age 17 to get married. At the time of her marriage, her family continued to grieve the sudden death of her twin sister 2 years before.

Sarah: This 30-year-old bookkeeper had been experiencing daily panic attacks for 4 months. Their onset had coincided with the one-year anniversary of her mother's death. Sarah had been pregnant when her mother died and had been afraid of having another miscarriage (she had already had two).

Michel: One of the two male members of the group, Michel was a 43-year-old plumber who had felt depressed for 7 months since separating from his wife of 14 years. He felt that the marital problems began 11 years ago when their son was born. His history revealed that within a year of his son's birth, Michel's father had died.

Kyle: The other male member of the group was a 36-year-old bartender. Kyle presented at the clinic after feeling depressed for 5 months with no identified precipitant. It was noted, however, that the onset of his depression coincided with his son's 10th birthday. When Kyle was 10, his mother had died.

Lois: The seventh member was a 29-year-old school teacher who complained of feeling lonely and isolated since her marital separation 3 years before.

THE BEGINNING STAGE

As elaborated in Chapter 5, STG therapists are confronted with many challenges. We consider many of these challenges unique to STG, reflecting both the nature of the patient population and the structure of the groups. The first clinical vignette emphasizes two foci of therapist interpretations that we believe are central to the therapist technique. Those foci involve the interpretation of transference phenomena and of patients' reactions to an absent member. Our discussion of the therapist's interventions represents guidelines for addressing the challenges confronted by the STG therapist.

The first session of the group, as with any new therapy group, elicited the theme of trust. In this case the theme was manifested by an atmosphere of "instant trust" whereby the group seemed to "jump start" any initial reluctance to self-disclose. They described their losses and identified with the similarities of each other's difficulties. One similarity involved their sense of isolation and ostracism from their respective social networks. They felt that no one had wanted to be involved in their grief. This ostracism was described in Chapter 3 as being a common experience of mourners, related to the twentieth century's societal wish to deny death and banish its icon. Several other similarities among the members were not discussed. These included the denial of the significance of the loss. For example, Margaret felt that she had "coped very well" with her previous losses. She had "kept on going" by adopting two children shortly after her fourth stillbirth. Similarly, Sarah had focused on her pregnancy rather than on the death of her mother. Although the significance of their losses had been denied, sadness was profoundly felt and expressed in this first session, with many members crying at various times. Their sadness revealed the sense of hopelessness and devastation common to this population.

The cohesive atmosphere of this first session was clearly attributable to the salient commonalities among the group members. Whereas this atmosphere of "instant trust" might be unusual for many new therapy groups, it is typical of the short-term loss groups of our program. The cohesiveness counteracted the anxiety common to initial group sessions, thus facilitating therapeutic process. However, this instant trust may have also reflected the members' tendency to deny distress and to adopt instead an attitude of "just keep on going." It may have reflected their wish to have trusting companions. The therapist offered her observation to the group that the similarities among them seemed to have created an atmosphere wherein they felt comfortable, safe, and understood.

As the session progressed, however, there was a sense of "waiting for the other shoe to drop." Although patients who have experienced loss typically want to feel close and intimate with someone, we have found that they are also frightened that such intimacy will render them vulnerable to possible criticisms, betrayals, and ultimately, to feeling even sadder when the group ends. As reviewed in Chapter 2, Bowlby's fourth variant of pathologic grief posits that "the bereaved . . . would avoid therapy and all other close relationships considering them a threat for the cherished secret (of denying the permanence of the loss)." To address the other side of the their wish to trust, therefore, the therapist offered her hypothesis that part of them may be wanting to "put the brakes on" lest they feel too vulnerable. There was some acknowledgment of feeling afraid of getting hurt again. As the first session drew to a close, the story surrounding each member's primary loss had been told, and they seemed to be wondering what to do next.

Six members returned for the second session. Ellen was absent. The session began with Alice noting that Ellen was absent. No one responded to this observation. Rather, there developed a discussion of the disadvantages of the various medications some of the members were taking. Although everyone became enthusiastically involved in this discussion, the topic of medications was off-task for a psychotherapy group for loss. The therapist attempted to focus the members on the group itself:

THERAPIST: I wonder if you're having a bit of the same concerns about the group. Certainly there's nothing tangible that you can sort of take in pill form, but you know, you do take your dosage of an hour and a half every week. And, so, maybe there are some concerns or fears that this cure is going to be worse than the anxiety or depression that brought you here; that in some way the side effects of this group are going to be worse than the concerns that brought you here.

Whereas all the group members had attended to the therapist's intervention, their discussion returned to the topic of medications. The emphasis had changed, however, in that only the positive aspects of medications were now being discussed. Their tenacity in discussing medications had two equally plausible yet somewhat contradictory implications for group process. Because medications were now being portrayed as positive and helpful, perhaps the members were implying that they did not need therapy after all and could thus abandon this anxiety-provoking experience of group therapy. Conversely, if the first interpretation had been accurate, that is, if they were using their discussion of the medications as a metaphor for their feelings about the group, then the patients were actually stating their hopefulness about the group. Furthermore, both sets of dynamics could have been operating simultaneously. In any case, they were still not directly discussing their losses, the group experience, or their feelings concerning either. They also were not directly responding to the therapist's intervention.

Since the patients neither confirmed nor disavowed the intervention, it was difficult for the therapist to assess its accuracy. This lack of response represents a common difficulty for the STG therapist and commonly evokes countertransferential feelings. The therapist may feel incompetent, inadequate, and unable to make an impact on the group. Such feelings may reflect a projective identification of the group in that regressive feelings of anger with earlier caretakers are being projected onto the therapist. This anger may stem from early neglect or rejection. As reviewed in Chapter 2, we believe that the group's reaction to the therapist's interpretation is consistent with the work of Bowlby, who postulated that the relationship of the mourner to the deceased is often marred by hostile dependency, angry possessiveness, and insecure attachment, which have their roots in childhood bereavement over repeated separations and rejections.

Another possible explanation for the patients' reaction to the therapist is that the groups take place in a hospital setting. Consequently, the therapist may be associated with the medical staff who failed to save their loved ones. As postulated in Chapter 3, survivors project angry feelings (which originated in ambivalence toward the lost loved one) onto caretakers, whom they blame for having been incompetent, negligent, and sloppy in their ministrations to the deceased. The therapist's difficulty is particularly disconcerting because his or her interventions are so often based on inference. In a short-term therapy group, the therapist cannot afford to accumulate substantial evidence before intervening. Nor can he or she allow the group to engage in lengthy defensive maneuvers. The therapist feels the time pressure and must rely on the courage of his or her convictions, and belief in a theoretical understanding of the patients' difficulties.

The session continued with Sarah talking about going to the dentist. The medications made it easier for her to sit in the chair without panicking or feeling trapped "for like, about an hour and a half while he drills away at you." The therapist ventured another interpretation:

THERAPIST: Well, I'm thinking that in some ways coming to this therapy group is like coming to the dentist's office in that for about an hour and a half, you're asked to open your mouth while I drill away at painful feelings and—

Margaret interrupted by saying "And we'd rather not." The rest of the members laughed. This section illustrates the evolution of the theme of faith in therapy. This theme probably emerged at this point because the members were beginning to trust each other enough to feel committed to the group, and they were beginning to feel intimate with each other. Conflicts associated with this theme include the wish that their risks will bring benefits versus their fear of more disappointments and failure. They looked to the therapist for reassurance. The therapist continued, focusing on their fears:

THERAPIST: Well, I think it is difficult for you. I'm sure you're wondering whether this group is going to be a bitter pill to swallow or whether it's going to help, or whether it might even make you worse.

Margaret nodded and spoke of how she had argued with her referring therapist about coming to the group. The argument involved her stating that she had dealt with the stillbirths of 20 years ago while the referring therapist pointed out that she was sobbing continually. She reluctantly agreed that she had some unfinished business in that area.

Responding to Margaret, the group continued with Sarah recounting the events of her mother's death. She had felt nothing at the time, and shortly thereafter she had focused on her newborn baby. At this point there was much discussion among the members concerning taking care of children and putting them first. Sarah remarked that her husband always needed her to take care of him, too. Everyone joined in at this point, jovially describing how they were surrounded by incompetent supervisors, bosses, spouses, for whom they must care. The mood had quickly changed from the sadness associated with Margaret's losses and the guilt hinted at by Sarah, to a jolly, and probably defensive one. The therapist attempted to put the group back on track by offering the following interpretation:

THERAPIST: So there seems to be a lot of protection going on. You take responsibility for other adults, covering up for them, always appearing calm and confident. I suspect, though, that there's also some resentment. You know, you take care of everyone else and when does it get to be your turn? And perhaps you would like that from me; that I take care of you in the way you've always wanted to be cared for and never have been. But then that might mean trusting me to be competent and capable of taking care of you, unlike the other people in your lives whom you've never been able to depend on. And I suppose also trusting that if you talk about the hurt and the pain that you have gone through, that somehow it will help rather than just making you feel worse.

Margaret responded first and talked about how she probably had been depressed for many years without realizing it. Alice and Michel agreed, describing how their children had interfered with their enjoyment of life. Sarah and Kyle joined in discussing their difficulties caring for children. Lois described how her students terrorized the school. While the patients were indeed discussing their resentment, it was being directed toward their children. They had originally been discussing incompetent supervisors, bosses, and spouses. The protection of these individuals was continuing. The therapist continued:

THERAPIST: I'm wondering if part of the reason this conversation about parents and children is coming up today is that in some ways, you know at the back of your mind, you're wondering what kind of parent I'm going to be with you. Perhaps you're worried that you're going to be a real handful of rambunctious kids for this single parent to handle and that you'll overwhelm me.

Margaret responded directly by saying to the therapist that "it would be nice if you looked after me—looked after my needs—but I don't expect that anyone really wants to." Michel agreed with this. Margaret continued, describing how she had gone to her family doctor wanting him to help her but that "there is no mommy out there." She continued in the same breath to describe how she had been very concerned about her new supervisor who "did not know the ropes." She explained: "Sometimes I feel I manipulate him to do what I know is right. I advise him but with these fellows and their big egos, you can't tell them what to do." This comment was an interesting association to the transference interpretation. Several of the members joined in this seemingly entertaining conversation of how stupid all authority figures are. Conversely, Margaret spoke of how her former supervisor had been very competent. She could be frank with him. She described a confrontation they had had shortly before his death. She acknowledged feeling very guilty about this and thought this was what had "set [her] off." The therapist responded with:

THERAPIST: I guess it might be difficult when you're in a role of being very responsible—you know all of you are—and you come into this group and you may not understand how I conduct the group. Maybe there's part of you that would fantasize about taking me aside and "showing me the ropes," to do the job the way you'd like to see it done. Maybe there's a fantasy that you'd like to lead the group yourselves. And I suppose it would be hard to tell me that directly, in case I up and died on you and then you'd feel guilty.

Sarah spoke sadly of how she remembered all the fights she had had with her mother before her death. Kyle spoke of fighting with his mother before her death. Alice recounted arguments with her twin sister before she had died. There was a feeling of profound guilt in the room.

According to Freud (1917/1957a), reproaches against the self in the melancholic are understood as being originally directed at the lost object. This is clearly shown in the above material. Bowlby (1963) has posited that when the anger becomes unconscious and displaced, be it toward the self or inappropriate objects, then the mourning becomes pathologic. As can be seen in the session, the patients' unconscious anger at their lost object is easily displaced onto the person of the therapist or the therapy itself. As they become more aware of these feelings, they again shift the anger back onto themselves in the familiar and less threatening form of self-reproach.

The therapist summarized the interchange between guilt and anger:

THERAPIST: So it is difficult to have a fight with someone, to get angry with someone or tell someone that you're disappointed with them if there's a possibility that they may die. And there'll be a lot of guilt afterwards. And maybe that's part of your difficulty in confronting me with how you feel about what I say or do in here; you're afraid you might hurt my feelings, or that I might not come back. Perhaps some of you are feeling guilty about Ellen not being here today. I wonder if your fantasy is that her absence has something to do with you.

Michel responded:

MICHEL: No, I think she didn't come back 'cause she didn't feel like she could talk in here. Like nobody asked her what she was crying about.

MARGARET: Yes, I did; I asked her if she was okay.

MICHEL: Well, yeah, but I mean like the therapist could have maybe asked her what was upsetting her, you know, brought her out more. Like I came here looking for the whys, the dos, the don'ts. She (the therapist) has not done a good job. See, so now I'm here to find my own answer.

SARAH: [*Interrupting*] I think it was just too much for Ellen, hearing everything, like when I was talking about my mother. She was really upset, you could just tell, you know. But she couldn't say anything. Then when she started crying, I thought, well, I guess, yeah, I thought you (the therapist) maybe should do something, like to calm her down, so she wouldn't feel so bad.

KYLE: Or maybe you (the therapist) should have stayed with her after group and not just stopping it right at 11:30.

SARAH: Yeah, I kinda wondered about that too, you know.

ALICE: [*Interrupting*] Well, I think she (the therapist) wouldn't be running the group if she, you know, she must know how you're supposed to do it, you know, get on with your life.

MARGARET: Well, I think she was overwhelmed by what I said. You know, I was kind of upset and maybe said too much.

MICHEL: I don't think it makes a difference how we feel about Helen (*sic*). I'm upset about my wife, not some stranger.

MARGARET: Yeah, I feel sort of annoyed, or frustrated with you (the therapist) 'cause how can you feel bad about losing someone you never even got to know?

LOIS: I think we need to get to know how to stop dwelling on the past, like how do we stop feeling like this.

THERAPIST: So there are some mixed feelings about me. There is some disappointment that I didn't take care of Ellen better, calm her down; that I point out that you may have some feelings about her not being here today. And there's the hope that I really do know what I'm doing, that I am going to help you.

They continued to discuss their fantasies about Ellen's absence. They imagined many scenarios. The therapist commented:

THERAPIST: There seem to be many fantasies about why Ellen is not here today. The common aspect of your fantasies is, however, that you were responsible in some way: You didn't talk to her enough; you put her on the spot too much; she couldn't handle hearing all about your mother; you overwhelmed her. And I'm wondering if this is a pattern for you all. That when someone goes away—even when they die—and you don't know "the whys," then you imagine that it has to have something to do with you—that fight you had just before the death.

There was a moment of silence after this interpretation. Slowly they began to acknowledge some anger that Ellen had not told them why she was absent. The therapist offered her hypothesis that there may also be some anger at other people who had left them in the past. The session ended with the emerging theme of how to express anger without hurting (killing) anyone.

The interchange of guilt and anger reflects the conflictual aspects associated with their wish to trust. These aspects include fears of being betrayed, attacked, and being incapable of overcoming their difficulties by themselves. Notice how quickly Margaret defended herself by stating that she had asked Ellen what she had been crying about. The guilt the group felt regarding Ellen's absence suggested that it was perhaps premature for the members to express their anger at Ellen for betraying their trust by not showing up. The therapist focused, therefore, on the interpretation of transference. By focusing on the transference relationship, the patients were encouraged to become aware of their expectations and disappointments concerning the therapist. Eventually they were able to get in touch with their expectations of her.

The wish seemed to be that she would be a helpful provider both within and outside of the group.

We have noted that there is often the hope that the therapist will provide the answers concerning what to talk about in the group, the grieving process, how to form new relationships and find happiness. In effect, the patients want the therapist to make life safe again and to gratify their frustrated dependency needs. Dependency on the therapist tends to be pronounced during the beginning stage, perhaps because many patients have had no previous group experience. On occasion, patients display their curiosity about the therapist by inquiring directly whether she or he has experienced a loss and how it was resolved. The importance of identifying the transference, especially the negative phenomena, is based on the assumption that loss patients attempt to substitute others, including the therapist, for their lost gratifying object (Chapter 2). Despite the substantial activity level of the therapist, negative transference phenomena seem to be elicited by the type of therapist activity that is predominantly interpretive and clarifying rather than directive and supportive.

The therapist addressed the negative transference by interpreting the frustrations and disappointments with her and the patients' fear of the same. By her interpreting the "unspeakable" the patients were indirectly encouraged by the therapist to express their "negative" feelings. The therapist's acceptance of these feelings is believed to have promoted an atmosphere of safety wherein ambivalence toward other important figures, especially the lost object(s), were explored. As reviewed in Chapter 2, we believe that it is the patients' intolerance of their ambivalent feelings towards the lost object that is etiologically related to pathologic grief, rather than the ambivalence per se. In this session we believe that it was the therapist's acceptance of their feelings that led to the willingness of the group members to disclose the arguments and fights that had occurred with the lost objects prior to their death and then to the discussion of their feelings toward the absent member, Ellen.

Whereas Alice began the session by commenting on Ellen's absence, the group did not address this for some time. It was as if they were afraid of "speaking ill of the dead." Eventually, they did share their fantasies concerning Ellen's absence. It is important to note that it was not known at that time whether Ellen would or would not be returning to the group. It was interesting, therefore, that all the patients assumed that she had dropped out. Although there were many fantasies concerning why Ellen had not returned, no one had fantasized that she chose to leave for her own reasons. The guilt was prevalent, and the patients' sense of responsibility was profound. Their anger was also present but that emotion was more difficult to acknowledge. Such difficulties tolerating and expressing anger are common to this population. Their reaction to the loss of Ellen was interpreted as being similar to their reactions to past losses. Identifying such here-and-now group behavior and linking this with past relationships are advocated in the STG technical approach. This linking is the crucial use of the "empty chair." Absenteeism is generally considered to have a demoralizing effect on psychotherapy groups. However, in STG for loss, we have found that absenteeism can be utilized very effectively to identify common patterns of reacting to loss. By the end of the session, the patients were slowly beginning to explore their misperceptions concerning past losses.

MIDDLE STAGE

The second vignette presents a session from the middle stage of this same loss group. The central theme is the recurring one of the patients' reaction to an empty chair. In this section, however, we focus on characteristic patient activity. We understand this activity as reflecting strategies and responses to the tasks and obstacles with which patients are presented in STG. One task which the patients are confronted with is to cope with the therapist's increasing frustration of their dependency needs by persisting with the interpretive approach. These interpretations seem to confuse the patients, who at times receive them as arcane and seemingly irrelevant. The members want support, advice, nurturance, and the fulfillment of their needs that were frustrated by past relationships. Because the therapist does not help by telling them what to do, the patients react by behaving as if the therapist is not needed. They turn to each other for advice, support, and ideas. They compare what has worked and what has not. They exchange advice freely, in contrast to the therapist whom they see as deliberately withholding information and solutions.

Pseudoindependent behavior occurs in an attempt to replace the group's need for the therapist. This pseudoindependence can take the form of ignoring not only the therapist's interpretations but also the therapist. The therapist often feels that he or she is superfluous. At such times, conversations between patients are devoid of affect and seem almost uninterruptable. Whereas patients may listen to the therapist's comments, they fail to respond or work with the interventions. They often react to transference interpretations as if the therapist were extremely self-centered or stupid. They ignore the suggestion that the therapist is in any way reminiscent of others from their past. Rather, they turn back to each other and resume their conversation where it was prior to being interrupted by the therapist's intervention. Their pseudoindependent stance can be seen as an attempt at mastery and autonomy, but it also reflects frustration. When the therapist refuses to comply with their wishes, the anger surfaces. The intensity of their anger reflects their reexperiencing of the loss of the original idealized object. These dynamics are illustrated in the following material.

The sixth session began with four members present. Kyle and Alice were absent. This was Alice's second (nonconsecutive) absence and Kyle's first. Ellen had been confirmed a dropout by session three.

(001) SARAH: Are we always in the same room?

LOIS: Yes.

[*Pause*]

SARAH: We're all dressed for winter.

(005) MARGARET: I wonder if it's still snowing?

SARAH: Quite a storm, eh?

[*Pause*]

MARGARET: Two missing.

[*Pause*]

(010) SARAH: Did you have a good week?

MARGARET: Yeah, I went to Red Deer and got stuck in the snow. So I had to spend an extra day, and miss a day of work [*Pretends to sob*].

[*Laughter*]

SARAH: It was funny 'cause when that snowstorm started, I brought
(015)   some work home, and the kids were in having a nap, and Tom was just watching the sports network, and I was working, and I had this little radio on so I could hear the news and it said the blizzard was going to miss us and I looked outside and it was so white you couldn't see anything! [*Laughing*] Yeah, really missed us!

(020) MARGARET: It was pretty bad, the motel we were in, the power went off in the middle of the night, and the power runs the water, so we had no heat, light, water, phone, radio, TV, but the water was the biggest thing. They brought us a pail to flush the toilet.

MICHEL: There was a lot of people who got abandoned out of town; I
(025)   bet a lot of people skiing.

MARGARET: I'm very glad I didn't get caught on the highway, sitting in the car. Some people sat there for 6 hours. I'd have had a nervous breakdown.

THERAPIST: Maybe the fantasy is that the two absent members are
(030)   snowbound somewhere and need to be rescued.

LOIS: We wouldn't know where to look! [*Laughter*] Besides, the highway patrol are really quite excellent at locating snowbound cars.

THERAPIST: Well, I'm wondering what your fantasies are about the fact that two members aren't here; how it makes you feel that they're
(035)   not here for you.

MARGARET: I don't expect people to be there for me, somehow. I just know I have to rely on myself. If I don't expect it, I'm not disappointed, I guess.

MICHEL: Yeah, it's better not to count on people, not expect anything,
(040)   not to need people, 'cause they do let you down.

MARGARET: Yeah, and I always forgive them—they have a good reason, they're not letting me down, they have a reason for not being here.

THERAPIST: And somehow the hope is that if you can understand why Kyle and Alice are not here today, then you won't feel what you
(045)   feel, which is worried, disappointed, hurt, perhaps angry.

MARGARET: Or if they were letting us down, letting the group down, it's something they couldn't help, they had a bad week . . .

SARAH: I agree.

MARGARET: That would be my worst fear for them, is that they had a
(050)   traumatic experience or time or something and they couldn't come. I think about them during the week. I guess we all do that.

SARAH: I think about Alice, because she seems to have so much going on in her life at one time, [*Lists Alice's concerns*]; a lot more than what I've got going on, you know?

(055) MARGARET: I almost feel guilty because I've been feeling so good lately!

LOIS: Me too, I've been feeling really good lately, too.

MARGARET: I was feeling really good when I got on the bus. I've been reading a book you recommended, Lois, about women who've suffered losses at childbirth; I became really sad really fast. But I
(060)   think it's a good book, people telling their experiences.

LOIS: But as the author points out, having one more child doesn't replace the loss.

MARGARET: Right. So I named all my babies. I never named the ones I lost.

(065) SARAH: How many did you have that you lost?

Margaret recounted the events surrounding each birth and death of her four lost children, fighting back the tears until she began to weep. Her sadness soon turned to anger at the medical staff:

MARGARET: But what I think about now is what the doctors did then
(070)   was just leave the baby, and I've often wondered, you know, Did they feed her? Did they give her water? She was such a beautiful baby. [*She begins to cry again.*] I guess this whole thing is helpful, because I guess, what I tried to do is replace each baby, 'cause I wanted two more babies, and . . . they were born very close . . .
(075)   [Recounts their birthdates] . . . So, I didn't really have time to grieve, I suppose I just got pregnant and thought, well fine, that's over, accept it.

SARAH: I know exactly how you feel about replacing because, well, I didn't carry a baby to term and then lose it, but I had a miscarriage.
(080)   But it's like right away, you're just thinking about the next pregnancy: I've got to get pregnant, I've got to get pregnant. It's really—

MARGARET: [*Interrupting*] I always thought it's too bad I didn't miscarry, why did I carry babies with abnormal defects so long—be-
(085)   cause often they say if it was a miscarriage, well, maybe there was something wrong with the baby, and you'd rather lose it than have a baby that was handicapped. I don't really understand what was wrong. Although those particular birth defects are common to my ethnic background, must be genetic. [*To Lois:*] So your book has
(090)   been really helpful . . .

Margaret continued to summarize the book's content with Sarah unsuccessfully attempting to introject the similarities with her own situation. Finally she succeeded in interrupting Margaret and recounted the story of her miscarriage, including her treatment by the medical staff:

(095) SARAH: And this intern had come in the night that I was brought in, he asked the usual questions and at that time I was smoking, and he told me that that's why I'm probably going to lose this baby . . . I was so upset, I told him I don't smoke four packs of cigarettes a day, just five cigarettes a day. For him to say that, I thought he was
(100)   really mean. I remember when he left, I just burst out crying. And nobody was there; I just waited for my doctor to come.

THERAPIST: This is something similar to what Margaret was saying:

feeling sort of guilty in some way, guilty that you couldn't provide
an atmosphere where these infants could develop, perhaps guilty,
(105)   you know, that something you did hurt or killed these babies.

SARAH: Yeah, that's a strong feeling.

MARGARET: Well, yeah, I had feelings of guilt. What did I do? Was it
the time I jumped over the fence, and you're not supposed to? But
it's probably genes.

(110) There was some discussion about other people they had known who
had had miscarriages or stillbirths. The theme evolved into how times
and the medical profession had changed:

LOIS: Well, I was watching this documentary on CBC [Canadian Broadcasting Corporation] or PBS [Public Broadcasting System] about
(115)   how doctors can now detect many of the various defects with the
use of amniocentesis and ultrasound. The thing is, of course, then
you have to decide whether to abort a handicapped child. That
point has been well documented in many of the journals I've read
on this subject.

(120) MARGARET: [Angrily] Well, I'm probably still very angry with the
whole medical profession, and nurses, and hospitals, because of
the treatment you receive after you've lost a baby. They put you
in a room with other mothers who have babies. . . . The next day
they brought me a baby and I said, "That's not mine," and she
(125)   argued with me. And they came around in the morning with little
packages of Ivory soap and samples of stuff. And they say "Are
you breast-feeding or bottle?"

The other members interjected as a chorus with remarks such as
"You're kidding!" "How awful!" "That's terrible!"

(130) MARGARET: I'd like to go and do something to reform the medical
profession—you know, like go inside the hospital and see if
they're doing things right and maybe if they're not, you know, I'd
like to campaign against them, and insist that they treat women .
. . .

(135) LOIS: Well, I certainly recommend to any women having children
nowadays to use a midwife. The labor tends to be shorter because
the woman is in a familiar environment, so she's calm and relaxed.
Natural childbirth has been shown to be much less traumatic for
the child, too.

(140) THERAPIST: Well, I guess you're talking about, on the one hand, your guilt—Did you do something wrong—and on the other hand, your anger at the medical profession: doctors, nurses who are very unfeeling, and in some ways sadistic. And I'm wondering whether there's a similarity with what happens in this group, with the two
(145) absent members today, if there are any feelings of guilt, something you did, that drove Alice and Kyle away and on the other hand, any feelings of anger at *this* medical professional for being somewhat sadistic or unfeeling in not telling you where they are, for not taking better care of them last week. There may even be some
(150) feelings of envy that they're snowbound in some ski resort while you're here having to work hard at facing painful feelings. So I wonder if there's any similarities between what you're feeling about past losses and what you're feeling today in this group, and whether you feel this group is miscarrying, in a way, in the sense
(155) that two of its children are not here today.

MARGARET: I was rather angry at the end of the last session because I felt we were skirting the issues always, myself included. I did feel that maybe Michel and—Lyle, is it?

LOIS: Kyle.

(160) MARGARET: Kyle, because they don't speak sometimes because myself or Alice, or you (Sarah), we talk so much.

MICHEL: It's no problem.

MARGARET: I just wonder how much help we are to you.

MICHEL: That's why I come to the session: any help I can get, or any
(165) new information, or anything, I guess it's all feelings.

SARAH: I don't even know what Kyle's problem is, what his loss is, does anybody know what his loss is?

[*Knock on door, Kyle arrives.*]

SARAH: Just talking about you!

(170) KYLE: I bet you were. Sorry I'm late, my worst anticipations have come true, one of the guys left work, so it's just gone nuts!

There are many questions about Kyle's work.

THERAPIST: So I guess it's difficult to say directly to Kyle the feelings you had when he wasn't here.

(175) [*Pause*]

SARAH: First, Margaret and I thought we were the only ones here, till we saw Michel walk by, then she goes: "Oh, there he goes."

MARGARET: We were speculating why you might not be here. I said the worst thing would be if you'd really had a traumatic experience (180) or were really down and couldn't come, because that reason to me would make me very sad.

KYLE: I think myself if I'd had, well, I've had panic attacks all week, in anticipation of this, I think, and today I feel really tense right now. Just coming here, being able to sit here with you for awhile, is good (185) for me. It's a little island of calm for me.

MARGARET: I think sometimes you hold yourself in because you don't want to let go in here, because will you be able to cope when you go back to work. I felt really depressed after the last session. I was wondering whether you and Michel were getting anything out of (190) it because you don't speak as much, and I was thinking, I speak too much.

SARAH: Me too.

KYLE: Well, for myself, I think it's much the same, it's just our nature to be quieter. I know I think a lot about what goes on in here. (195) Though I may not say much while I'm here, it does help.

THERAPIST: Margaret, you changed how you were feeling—originally you said you were angry and you changed it to depression. And though I'm sure there is a link between your depression and your anger, maybe what's harder to say is that you're angry at Kyle and (200) Michel for what you don't get from them, rather than what you don't give to them, the fact that you don't hear what they're thinking, what they're feeling, and I guess it's more difficult again to express being angry at members of this group.

MARGARET: Maybe. I guess I was feeling, you know, What's this group, (205) is it helping me? I hadn't expressed how I felt last week, so I was hoping I could express more how I feel this week, because it helps you when you can say how you feel.

THERAPIST: It's also very frightening, from what we're hearing. Fearing that, if you were to express how you feel, even though we've heard (210) it does make you feel better, I think you're afraid you won't be able to stop crying, and we've talked about this before, to express anger means you become homicidal. If you express sadness, you won't stop crying, you'll float away in your own tears. So while it may be particularly true for Kyle, I think all of you have the fear that (215) stops you from expressing the feelings you have for each other, and about the people in your past.

KYLE: Is it normal to linger on the loss for years, or something like that?

LOIS: Well, people go through stages of mourning in different time frames—

(220) KYLE: [*Sarcastically*] Is that so, Dr. Lois?

THERAPIST: Well, Lois, I think you want to help the others by giving them a better understanding of what they're all going through. I wonder if perhaps you feel sort of scared by all the anger and sadness in the room, and that by offering a rational understanding
(225) of what's going on, perhaps the feelings will go away. And I don't think you're the only one who is scared by these feelings, there is certainly a real need to try and get some meaning or explanations for what happened, the deaths, and for what you are all feeling.

Margaret interrupts by talking about how she cared for her son's kids
(230) when his wife was having another baby.

THERAPIST: My hunch is, Margaret, that you are sort of being in the role of surrogate mother here as well. What I mean by that is that you sort of protect the group, you sort of express that you're a little bit angry, and you were angry with Kyle and Michel for not talking.
(235) But at the same time you don't push them, and you sort of protect them by not pursuing that line. Michel said a little bit about his father. And now that Kyle sounded angry with Lois, you intervene again, the peace keeper, by talking about yourself and getting them off the hook. My hunch is that the role of mother is quite
(240) familiar to you, and in a sense you take it in this group too, and of course, the group allows you to do that.

MARGARET: [*To Michel*] When did you lose your father?

Michel recounts the death of his father and the estrangement from his wife. There is a discussion about whether death or divorce is easier to
(245) cope with.

THERAPIST: Well, you're sort of saying that with the separation the hope remains, and that that ambiguity is more difficult to deal with, and that you have many mixed feelings about your wife. I think, though, that those mixed feelings are there with the deaths as well.
(250) You know we've heard about the sadness, the guilt, I'm sure some relief that, you know, those children did not live. So though it may be easier to see after a separation, I think there are a lot of mixed feelings after a death, including anger at being alone.

MICHEL: Well, yes.

(255) SARAH: I think I was mad at my mom too, because she was sick a long time before she was even diagnosed with cancer, and she wouldn't go to the doctor: "No, I have to go to work, I have to go to work." So there, so run yourself into the ground, but heaven forbid you go to the doctor, you know? It really made me mad.

(260) MARGARET: Maybe she had to go to work to cope with—

SARAH: [*Interrupting*] I don't know, she was—

LOIS: [*Interrupting louder*] Work can be therapeutic—

SARAH: [*Interrupting even louder*] She didn't know what was wrong—

MARGARET: Work can be an escape, you know.

(265) THERAPIST: I think it's difficult to hear Sarah's anger at her mother.

Sarah continues to express anger with her mother but quickly changes her focus to her anger with her father:

SARAH: I phoned and my dad said, "Oh, we took mother to the hospital last night." You know, he didn't even phone me and tell me (270) anything was wrong. I'd phone every week and ask him, "Is it cancer?" And he'd say, "Oh, no."

Sarah continues describing her father's response to the various hospitalizations and tests conducted on her mother as one whereby she was kept in the dark.

(275) THERAPIST: So even though your father wanted to protect you, he actually hurt you more by not allowing you time to prepare for your mother's death. And I'm wondering if there's a message in there for me: that perhaps I'm trying to protect you from news about Alice by not telling you where she is, but then I'm not (280) allowing you time to prepare for her "death" from this group. I guess it's difficult to confront me with your anger that I'm not telling you in much the same way you protect your dad from your anger that he didn't tell you about your mum.

MARGARET: I keep forgetting about her.

(285) MICHEL: When you bring it up all the time, I get worried.

MARGARET: Each time you bring it up, I realize that since she's not here I'm just not going to think about her.

SARAH: But what's worse, blocking it out—

KYLE: Or talking about it?

(290) LOIS: Or tormenting yourself all the time.

MARGARET: Well, you talk about anger, I have felt such great anger.

Margaret described what had happened when she went for tests during the 8th month of her fifth pregnancy. No one would tell her any of the results until finally the doctor came and told her the fetus was (295) encephalic.

MARGARET: After I heard, I foolishly took the bus—I don't know why I don't take taxis in moments of crises in my life—and I started to cry, and I'm sitting there, pregnant and crying, and the whole bus is, "Are you alright?" and I said, "I'm fine." And I remember (300) thinking, this was probably the year they were talking about God being dead, and I thought, if He isn't dead, I'll kill Him!

SARAH: That's an awful lot of anger.

THERAPIST: It was Alice that triggered your memory. I think that the connection is that you're probably angry with me, for not protect- (305) ing Ellen first, and then Alice; not being a good enough mum to hold this family together, and again, it's difficult to confront me with your anger. In much the same way you can't confront your father, your mother, the other people in your life who've let you down; that rational side of your mind which is stopping yourself (310) from expressing the feelings you're feeling. And it must, partly, be anger.

MARGARET: Maybe it's my anger at Alice; she should've been able to come here today. I worry about her because she mentioned suicide and although she said she'd never consider it, I still find it scary. (315) If she does, I'll be mad.

KYLE: How can you express your anger at someone who is dead? You really can't go out and stand at the grave site and yell and scream, it doesn't help. It's not a confrontation.

MARGARET: I don't even have a grave site for my babies. They just burn (320) them in the incinerator. . . . The thing is, I didn't want my first son, I wasn't married, I was very young. But I wouldn't consider abortion.

There is a discussion about abortion and large families. Margaret then opens her purse and hands out mints.

(325) SARAH: I think I was mad at my mom just because she never told me the truth. Even when I'd phone her, you know, and nobody else

would phone me and say, you know, Mom's really sick, she's losing a lot of weight, she's really weak, she can't get out of bed anymore, and nobody did. It was like, when she got admitted to
(330)   the hospital the last time, she was in there for three or four days before my dad even phoned. He didn't even phone me, I phoned!

MARGARET: Did he think you'd have trouble accepting it?

SARAH: Oh, yeah. He'd start walking to see her, because that's where my mom used to work, to pick her up!

(335) MARGARET: He'd forget.

SARAH: He'd forget! And then he said he'd remember and then he'd be really disoriented, like, Where should I go? Where is there to go? I was just expecting him to fall apart.

MICHEL: You can't get angry with your mom, because she's not there
(340)   to be angry with, you can't get angry with your dad.

SARAH: And the thing is, with bowel cancer, it's 99 percent curable if it's caught in time. So that's why I was so upset. She had gone months and months without going to the doctor. She was supposed to go every 6 months for her blood pressure pills. She'd
(345)   phone up and say, I'm too busy at work, and the doctor would call in the repeat prescriptions! And I think I was mad at my dad. Even now I can't talk about my mom to my dad. I start talking about it and I see in his face all the pain, and I just can't say: I was pissed off at you, I was pissed off at you for months.

(350) MARGARET: Sounds like you're mad at your dad, or mad at yourself.

SARAH: Well, I think that a lot of times when I phoned, I'd want to ask my mom exactly what was going on, but because she didn't want to bring it up, I didn't want to. You know, what do you say? So did you lose ten pounds? Are you sicker? You can't say that to
(355)   someone who's dying of cancer!

THERAPIST: We'll continue next week.

This sixth session of the group depicts patient behavior that we have found to be characteristic of the loss groups. The session began with much tension. Indeed, as Sarah pointed out, the anxiety began in the waiting room where she and Margaret believed they were the only two members present (176–177). In part, we believe that the tension was attributable to the empty chairs of Kyle and Alice. Our belief is supported by the way in which the session began. Sarah asked: "Are we always in the same room?" (001), perhaps reflecting her desire that the absent members would be able to find the group. Shortly thereafter

Margaret noted that there were "Two missing" (008). Margaret and Sarah attempted to dissipate the tension by joking about the storm (004–023). The therapist's intervention (029–030) attempted to overcome this distraction by focusing the group on the absent members. Lois further distracted the group by providing a rational reassurance that the highway patrol are competent (031–032). Again the therapist intervened, maintaining her focus on the absent members (033–035). The tentative style associated with her second attempt reflected, perhaps, that she was rather daunted by the strength of the group's defensiveness. Margaret and Michel finally responded to this intervention by explaining the rationale behind their defensiveness (036–042). Their response allowed the therapist to interpret their defense of rationalization (043–045).

Sarah hinted that Alice's absence was related to the previous session by recounting Alice's many difficulties (052–054). Sarah's account triggered some survivor guilt in Margaret: "I almost feel guilty because I've been feeling so good lately!" (055). Margaret's association to her survivor guilt was to the death of her children (057–139). While Margaret engaged in work at this point, she also rescued the group from exploring their feelings regarding Alice. Indeed, the group did not return to discussing Alice until much later (284) after being prompted by the therapist's interpretation (275–283). Even at that point, the topic was quickly deflected, again by Margaret discussing the death of her fifth child (291–301). Undaunted, the therapist persisted with her focus on Alice (303–311). Finally the defensiveness gave way:

MARGARET: Maybe it's my anger at Alice; she should've been able to come here today. I worry about her because she mentioned suicide and although she said she'd never consider it, I still find it scary. If she does, I'll be mad. (312–315)

It is interesting to speculate whether Margaret's concern over the absent members that she had voiced earlier—" . . . my worst fear . . . is that they had a traumatic experience or time or something and they couldn't come. . . ." (049–051)—actually represented a projection of her anger at the absent members. Margaret's acknowledgment of her anger at Alice (312) led to Kyle acknowledging the depths of his anger—" . . . stand at the grave site and yell and scream . . . " (317)—and Margaret's acknowledgment of her anger at the child who died: "I didn't want my first son, I wasn't married . . . " (320–321). Sarah's exploration of her anger toward her mother, who died of bowel cancer (325–355) is perhaps the most poignant of the three acknowledgments and represents an important work phase for her.

The middle section of this session represents a pathway between survivor guilt (055) and anger at the deceased (312). First, Margaret's survivor guilt was transformed into sadness over the losses (059), which in turn was quickly transformed into anger at the medical profession (069). Throughout their tirades against the medical profession, the patients hinted at their guilt vis-à-vis the deceased (083–139). Theoretically, their anger and their guilt are understood as the displacement of anger at the deceased for having abandoned them. The therapist attempted to interpret the various facets of this progression from survivor guilt to anger at the deceased and to link this to the here-and-now group situation (140–155). Whereas the therapist's interpretation did integrate all the themes of the session, it reflects, perhaps, a danger for the STG therapist: succumbing to the temptation to interpret everything that occurs in these dense, accelerated sessions in one overloaded interpretation.

Following her interpretation, the members were not yet ready to discuss Alice. The focus shifted to Kyle, the other absent member. Margaret stated that she had been angry at the end of the previous session owing to the defensiveness of the members and the silence of Michel and Kyle (156–161). However, she later disavowed her anger, describing her feeling as one of concern that she was monopolizing the group (188–191). Margaret's confrontation of Michel (163) was diverted by Sarah expressing her anger at Kyle, a safer target because he was absent (166–167). With uncanny timing, Kyle arrived at that very moment (168). The group's attention shifted to the more tenuous member, Kyle. With encouragement from the therapist (173–174; 196–203), the patients were able to begin to confront Kyle and Michel with their feelings toward them. With Kyle's and Michel's response to that confrontation, Sarah began to speak of her anger at her mother (255–259). Margaret and Lois succeeded in diverting this account (260–264), and Sarah began to discuss her anger at her father instead of at her mother (268–271). We understand this discussion as a displacement of the anger with the mother onto the father. As mentioned previously, this was where the therapist intervened (275–283) successfully, using a transference interpretation to return the focus to Alice for the final section of the session.

PATIENT ROLES

The patients' behavior is, in part, their response to the tension created by the therapist's role and other anxiety-provoking aspects of this session. Their response can be conceptualized as the formation of patient roles. We use the term *role* to refer to a well-defined set of behaviors presented by a patient that represents a conflict shared by other patients. Only part of the conflict, for example, the wish, may be obvious from the behaviors presented during a particular time interval. The behaviors, being compromise formations of the conflict, may appear to belong only to the patient occupying the role. Indeed, the other patients may attribute such behaviors (and conflict) only to that patient who continues to take a complementary position vis-à-vis the group. We have assigned labels to the patients who occupy the roles. It should be noted that either gender may occupy the roles described.

The emergence of a role is precipitated by a period of heightened anxiety associated with a particular conflict. Some patient roles emerge as if to fulfill what is wished for by the therapist, or what is defended against, while others emerge to fulfill other needs of the group. Each patient role is seen as serving both a defensive and an adaptive function. A role can be defensive in that it distracts the members from some anxiety-provoking material. A role can be adaptive in that on occasion all members need to defend themselves from anxiety-provoking material. For example, the survival of the group may require a "timeout" from overwhelming material. In addition, the various roles tend to help the group survive by gratifying regressive dependency needs. The emergence of a role may act to signal to the therapist that the group is attempting to procure a decrease in anxiety or an increase in support. To expect all members to engage in therapeutic work at all times is unrealistic. Nevertheless, these roles may interfere with the work of the group by preventing the occupier and the other group members from experiencing other aspects of themselves.

Our way of conceptualizing patient roles has implications for the therapist's technique. Because we conceptualize roles as reenacting shared conflicts, we interpret the hypothesized components of the conflicts as being common to all members. The therapist helps members identify and own that which they would prefer to project onto another group member. We also believe that when a patient occupies a particular patient role, she or he unwittingly serves a defensive function for the entire group. Therefore, when addressing a patient role, the therapist interprets to the group that all members are being rescued by the role occupier who permits them to disavow ownership of shared feelings and thoughts. Yalom (1985) has tended to focus more upon the defensive aspects of patient roles. The roles he has identified (e.g., the monopolizer) have been conceptualized as representing "problem" patients. From our perspective, the roles that emerge in STG reflect conflicts shared by all group members. The emergence of each particular patient role is congruent with a group theme. The following section summarizes our clinical observations concerning these roles in general, and in the illustrated group in particular.

The Apparition

"Now you see her, now you don't" characterizes the behavior of the apparition in the group. Often, she has come late to the first session with her attendance continuing to be erratic thereafter, with absenteeism, lateness, or early departure. In this group Alice had occupied the role of the apparition. This was the second session she had missed. Throughout this session the group seemed to react to her as if she were a confirmed dropout. The next candidate to occupy that role was Kyle.

The apparition typically offers reasonable excuses such as work schedules or illnesses as being responsible for her tardiness or absenteeism. Initially, the group is accepting of her excuses, often coming to her defense when she is confronted by the therapist:

MARGARET: Yeah, and I always forgive them—they have a good reason, they're not letting me down, they have a reason for not being here (041–042). . . . Or, if they were letting us down, letting the group down, it's something they couldn't help, they had a bad week . . . (046–047)

Similarly, they deny having any feelings toward the "empty chair."

MARGARET: I keep forgetting about her.

MICHEL: When you bring it up all the time, I get worried.

MARGARET: Each time you bring it up, I realize that since she's not here I'm just not going to think about her.

SARAH: But what's worse, blocking it out—(284–288)

Eventually the group begins to recognize the disruptive nature of this patient role as disclosures are interrupted or need to be repeated owing to the apparition's arrival.

With her continuing disappearances, the patients begin to acknowledge feeling confused by their inability to decide which is the appropriate emotion to be feeling and their desire not to "waste" an emotion before knowing whether it is justified. Their confusion reflects their assumption that an emotion has to be justified in order to be permitted. It also indicates that they have a variety of feelings with respect to the apparition. Through the therapist's interpretations of the censorship of their feelings as a defensive process, the group members begin to voice some feelings toward the "empty chair."

THERAPIST: And somehow the hope is that if you can understand why Kyle and Alice are not here today, then you won't feel what you feel, which is worried, disappointed, hurt, perhaps angry. (043–045)

Feelings of concern, sadness, regret, and guilt seem somehow easier to tolerate and own than those of frustration, anger, envy, or relief.

The "Is she in or is she out?" behavior of the apparition epitomizes ambivalence with respect to group membership. We wish to emphasize, however, that all group patients struggle with ambivalent feelings about remaining in the group. For loss patients, ambivalence represents a salient conflict and is therefore more pronounced in STG. The theme of ambivalence is common throughout the life of the group. Conflicts associated with this theme include the wish to belong and feel part of the group versus the wish to escape feeling trapped, vulnerable, and anxious. When addressing the apparition in the group, the therapist hypothesizes that she, the apparition, is enacting the group's ambivalence. Hence, the group's acceptance and defense of the apparition's disappearances are interpreted as representing the group's wish to disown their ambivalence while projecting it onto her. The behavior of the apparition is interpreted, therefore, as reflecting the entire group's fear of group commitment. It is also interpreted that the group is living vicariously through the apparition:

THERAPIST: There may even be some feelings of envy that they're snowbound in some ski resort while you're here having to work hard at facing painful feelings. (149–151)

In actuality the apparition does present the group with an ambiguous situation: Is she in or is she out? This ambiguity evokes ambivalence regarding whether or not to continue investing in the patient. The ambiguity surrounding the question of whether the apparition is lost or not can be reminiscent of the ambiguity associated with separations and divorces. As the group members begin to express their feelings toward the apparition, the therapist can link the here-and-now issue of ambivalence to the various conflicts evoked by the previous losses that brought patients into the group—for example, wishes for guarantees before risking intimacy, or fears of getting close only to be hurt if the person leaves.

By discussing the apparition's wish to abandon the group, the patients have the opportunity to speak their minds and to say goodbye in a way that was often denied them with regard to past losses:

MARGARET: We were speculating why you might not be here. I said the worst thing would be if you'd really had a traumatic experience or were really down and couldn't come, because that reason to me would make me very sad. (178–181)

Hence each patient can address the unspoken feelings and the unfinished business that haunt them from past losses. If the apparition's ambivalence results in her departure from the group, the therapist can continue to link the here-and-now loss with past losses by noting the similarity in the feelings elicited by the dropout: guilt (drove them away), anger (feeling abandoned), sadness (loss), relief (tension dissipated):

THERAPIST: Well, I guess you're talking about, on the one hand, your guilt—did you do something wrong?—and on the other hand, your anger at the medical profession: doctors, nurses who are very unfeeling and in some ways sadistic. And I'm wondering whether there's a similarity with what happens in this group, with the two absent members today, if there are any feelings of guilt, something you did, that drove Alice and Kyle away and on the other hand, any feelings of anger at *this* medical professional for being somewhat sadistic or unfeeling in not telling you where they are, for not taking better care of them last week. There may even be some feelings of envy that they're snowbound in some ski resort while you're here having to work hard at facing painful feelings. So I wonder if there's any similarities between what you're feeling about past losses and what you're feeling today in this group, and whether you feel this group is miscarrying, in a way, in the sense that two of its children are not here today. (140–155)

The departure of the apparition elicits the theme of survivor guilt:

MARGARET: I almost feel guilty because I've been feeling so good lately!

LOIS: Me too, I've been feeling really good lately, too. (055–056)

Conflicts associated with this theme include regrets about not having done more by including the dropout in the group activities. Patients may express wishes that they had said something differently. Fears about having said the wrong thing and regrets about being open or confrontive are commonly heard. It is unusual that the patients' fantasies include the idea that the dropout chose to leave for his or her own reasons. By leaving the empty chairs in the circle, the therapist insures there is a constant reminder of all other empty spaces in the patients' lives. This theme is again linked to each patient's original losses. After the apparition has resolved her ambivalence, one way or another, the group is more able to shift into a work phase (063–082; 312–355).

The Monk

Another patient role that is demonstrated in this middle session is that of the monk. This role is characterized by "a vow of silence." In the first part of this session, Michel enacts this role. He dutifully attends each session, is attentive to the other patients, yet remains silent. When invited to participate, the monk typically reassures the group that he is feeling better just by listening to the group's discussion and that he agrees with most of what has been said:

MICHEL: It's no problem (162) . . . That's why I come to the session: any help I can get, or any new information, or anything, I guess it's all feelings.(164–165)

Because Kyle arrived at that point (168), Kyle soon assumed the role.

KYLE: Well, for myself, I think it's much the same, it's just our nature to be quieter. I know I think a lot about what goes on in here, though I may not say much while I'm here, it does help. (193–195)

It is interesting to note that Kyle fluctuated between enacting the roles of apparition and monk in this group. The shift of roles for a single patient is consistent with our belief that roles do not represent the unique conflicts of a particular patient but functions required by the entire group. Typically the group does not challenge the monk. For example, Margaret stated: "I just wonder how much help we are to you" (163). Rather, the theme of intimacy tends to emerge. This theme is often accompanied by anger and guilt:

MARGARET: I was rather angry at the end of the last session, because I felt we were skirting the issues always, myself included. I did feel that maybe Michel and . . . Kyle, because they don't speak . . . (156–160) . . . wondering whether you and Michel were getting anything out of it because you don't speak as much and I was thinking, I speak too much. (189–191)

Ultimately the risk is that the entire group can become silent.

Conflicts associated with this theme include the fantasy that intimacy need not require the risk of vulnerability. It is this fantasy that is demonstrated so powerfully by the monk's silence:

KYLE: Just coming here, being able to sit here with you for awhile, is good for me. It's a little island of calm for me. (184–185)

Motivating this defensive fantasy is the fear of speaking in the group. This fear seems to be associated with the patient's anticipation of criticism and judgment, suggesting that there is guilt over some seemingly unspeakable wrongs that he has committed. Another possibility is the fear that spontaneous disclosure may open a Pandora's box of emotion that would overwhelm the speaker or the entire group:

MARGARET: I think sometimes you hold yourself in because you don't want to let go in here, because will you be able to cope when you go back to work. (186–188)

Hence the monk is permitted to sit in silence:

THERAPIST: Margaret, you changed how you were feeling—originally you said you were angry and you changed it to depression . . . maybe what's harder to say is that you're angry at Kyle and Michel for what you don't get from them, rather than what you don't give to them, the fact that you don't hear what they're thinking, what they're feeling, and I guess it's more difficult again to express being angry at members of this group. (196–203)

It is assumed that all group patients struggle with their fear of being judged and of becoming overwhelmed by emotion. Accordingly, the members would avoid delving into painful issues by believing that "time heals all." When addressing the monk in the group, the therapist hypothesizes that this patient's behavior is enacting the group's fears of being judged and of losing control:

THERAPIST: It's also very frightening, from what we're hearing. Fearing that, if you were to express how you feel, even though we've heard it does make you feel better, I think you're afraid you won't be able to stop crying, and we've talked about this before, to express anger means you become homicidal. If you express sadness, you won't stop crying, you'll float away in your own tears. *So while it may be particularly true for Kyle, I think all of you have the fear that stops you from expressing the feelings you have for each other, and about the people in your past.* (208–216)

In addition to diffusing the projective aspect of roles, interpretations made at the group level may also enhance group cohesion. Members realize the commonality of their fears, and thus their sense of isolation diminishes. Conversely, these interpretations may disrupt group cohesion. Members may resist identifying with others who display those very aspects that they themselves are trying to disown.

The Professor

The professor, enacted by Lois, offers an academic, intellectualized presentation of loss. She speaks in generalities, presenting parables and clichés to the group. She often cites self-help books, radio talk show guests, and so forth:

LOIS: the highway patrol are really quite excellent at locating snowbound cars (031–032). . . . But as the author points out, having one more child doesn't replace the loss (061–062). . . . Well, I was watching this documentary on CBC [Canadian Broadcasting Corporation] or PBS [Public Broadcasting System] about how doctors can now detect many of the various defects with the use of amniocentesis and ultrasound. The thing is, of course, then you have to decide whether to abort a handicapped child. That point has been well documented in many of the journals I've read on this subject (113–119). . . . Well, I certainly recommend to any women having children nowadays to use a midwife. The labor tends to be shorter because the woman is in a familiar environment, so she's calm and relaxed. Natural childbirth has been shown to be much less traumatic for the child, too (135–139). . . . Well, people go through stages of mourning in different time frames. (218–219)

It is rare that she discloses anything about personal loss(es). She seems to want a syllabus and a logical progression for the group. In effect, she demands guarantees from the therapist that the group will "work." The professor can present a formidable challenge to the therapist by competing for leadership. Indeed she seems to emerge to fulfill the wished-for role of the therapist who could explain logically and rationally everything they were feeling and experiencing. She frequently contradicts and discounts all therapist interventions, countering every interpretation with an alternative explanation. This tends to dilute the impact of interpretation on the patients. The rest of the members tend to sit back and watch the contest. The professor enacts the wish that the losses and the therapy will have meaning without uncertainty and be understandable without ambiguity. The professor's behavior also reflects the fear of emotionality by rationalizing that if only she could understand feelings, then they would become either permissible or unnecessary. In addition, she takes a passive–aggressive stance by indirectly challenging the competence of the therapist's leadership. It is hypothesized that anger toward the medical profession for not being competent enough to save the loved one(s) is also reenacted in the professor's provocations. This anger cannot be directly expressed, however, owing to the group's dependency on the medical profession and its representative, the therapist.

We hypothesize that conflicts associated with the themes of dependence on and confidence in the therapist are common to all group patients. The professor is understood to enact the conflicts for the entire group. The group's collusion with her challenge to the therapist's manner of conducting the group is reflected in their failure to confront the professor. Hence, the therapist interprets the various components of the conflict as belonging to all group members:

THERAPIST: Well, Lois, I think you want to help the others by giving them a better understanding of what they're all going through. I wonder if perhaps you feel sort of scared by all the anger and sadness in the room, and that by offering a rational understanding of what's going on, perhaps the feelings will go away. *And I don't think you're the only one who is scared by these feelings; there is certainly a real need to try and get some meaning or explanations for what happened, the deaths, and for what you are all feeling.* (221–228)

The Professional Nurturer

The professional nurturer emerges as if to fulfill the nurturing functioning that the group so wishes of the therapist. Margaret fulfills this role in the group. She is the patient who often brings gum or mints to the sessions and offers them to everyone including the therapist. She is soothing and seems capable of identifying with every experience mentioned in the group. In fact, she tends to monopolize the group, adeptly diverting all anxiety-provoking topics and "rescuing" emotionally distressed members. For example, in section 083–090, although Margaret was working hard at understanding her own losses, she interrupted Sarah to do so and failed to yield to Sarah's various attempts to join the discussion.

The professional nurturer competes with the therapist in terms of the group members' conscious or unconscious fantasies about how to behave as a therapist: She is openly supportive of group members, dismissing any attempt to explore their own contribution to the problems. Similarly, she tends to immediately deny all interpretations of negative transference. The professional nurturer seems to enact a perversion of the golden rule in that she "gives unto others what she wants others to give unto her." In other words, her primary motive is to receive rather than to give; she desperately wants to be taken care of. She also has very definite ideas about what the other has to do to satisfy her desires, although these are seldom verbalized. Disappointment is inevitable and tends to reinforce the fear that no one is either competent or caring enough to take care of her. The professional nurturer tends to be compulsively self-reliant and extremely resentful of that fact. The therapist addresses the role of the professional nurturer in the group by interpreting that all the patients want to be cared for and to receive unconditional acceptance. In addition, the therapist hypothesizes that rather than being "nice" to those who disappoint their needs, the patients would really like to rage against them. Their feelings of hurt and anger with respect to this neglect are disguised as altruism. The defensive aspect of "peace at all costs" is interpreted:

THERAPIST: Margaret, you changed how you were feeling—originally you said you were angry and you changed it to depression. And though I'm sure there is a link between your depression and your anger, maybe what's harder to say is that you're angry at Kyle and Michel for what you don't get from them, rather than what you don't give to them, the fact that you don't hear what they're thinking, what they're feeling, and I guess it's more difficult again to express being angry at members of this group. (196–203)

And later, the defensive role that Margaret plays for the group is interpreted:

THERAPIST: My hunch is, Margaret, that you are sort of being in the role of surrogate mother here as well. What I mean by that is that you sort of protect the group, you sort of express that you're a little bit angry, and you were angry with Kyle and Michel for not talking. But at the same time you don't push them, and you sort of protect them by not pursuing that line. Michel said a little bit about his father. And now that Kyle sounded angry with Lois, you intervene again, the peace keeper, by talking about yourself and getting them off the hook. My hunch is that *the role of mother is quite familiar*

to you, and in a sense you take it in this group too, and of course, the
group allows you to do that. (231–241)

ADDITIONAL PATIENT ROLES

We have identified two other patient roles that tend to emerge in the
short-term groups. They were not represented in the sessions
illustrated in this chapter. They are the Emotional Conductor and the
Cruise Director.

The Emotional Conductor

This patient role emerges when the group is struggling with the
"correct" way to emote. The emotional conductor is typically a weeper
or a pugilist. In other words, she tends to have a monopoly on a
particular emotion, which is usually sadness or anger. In effect, she
carries that emotion for the group. She also tends to prevent other
emotions from being experienced by the group: When these threaten
to emerge, she adeptly reinstates her (and their) preferred emotional
climate. At the same time, she tends to act as if there is no cerebral
cortex in that the presentation is purely emotional, almost devoid of
intellect and understanding. There is a lack of integration between the
various emotions as well as a lack of integration between emotion and
intellect. In addressing the role of the emotional conductor, the therapist interprets her contribution as a protection of the group and of
herself. In addition, the therapist emphasizes that all group patients
experience all kinds of emotions at various times and sometimes at the
same time. When addressing the emotional conductor the goal is to get
the patients to begin to experience their own affects and express them
in their own individual ways.

The Cruise Director

The cruise director is very witty, with lots of jokes and scathing
sarcasm. He tends to break the tension and thereby attempts to
"rescue" other members. He does, however, often unwittingly suggest
the transference issues although interpretations of transference are
overtly denied. He is also the one most likely to suggest going for coffee
after the group, or a postgroup barbecue. Hence he enacts the wish of
avoiding the gravity of the losses—past, present, and future, in their
lives. In addressing the role of the cruise director, the therapist inter-

prets his diversions as representing the defensive processes of the entire group. The therapist interprets the wish to turn the heavy work of therapy into a party that need never end.

TOWARD THE TERMINATION STAGE

The sixth session marks the mid-point of the group, evoking the theme of mortality. Conflicts associated with this theme include the wish for continued intimacy and depth versus the dread of termination. The patients attempt to avoid further intimacy by maintaining the group content on a rather superficial and more supportive level. The patients rationalize that there is no point in becoming closer because that would only increase the feeling of loss when the group ends. Despite the group's resistance, the therapist persists with here-and-now interpretations. He or she might also suggest that the members are angry with the therapist, who will "pull the plug" on the group by ending it. We consider that the focus on transference is therapeutic and central. The rationale for this focus includes the idea that if the patients can tolerate their disappointment in the transference relationship, they then may begin to tolerate the imperfection of other relationships. Although there is an intense resistance to intimacy, an "all for one" attitude does prevail as individual patients "agree" to continue working as a group and enter the second half of therapy. The patients become increasingly concerned for and interested in each other, risking more intimacy. Feelings of acceptance and closeness by the group members toward each other become progressively more evident as therapy continues. At the same time, the underlying affects of sadness and anger with respect to the loss are voiced in the group. Each session is full and the 90 minutes generally pass very quickly.

To recognize and talk about their underlying feelings can be very frightening for patients. Often their affects have been suppressed for years. By finally acknowledging these feelings, patients frequently voice their fear of being overwhelmed by intense reactions once their defenses are relaxed. Some patients have been taught by their families that, particularly when dealing with the dead, anger is inappropriate. They often feel that the memory of the departed must be honored. Hence, they learn "If you cannot say anything nice, then do not say anything at all." The anger at the loss is often intellectualized or denied by emphasizing that the deceased did not choose to abandon the bereaved. Often, patients will persist with this emphasis despite the death's having been precipitated or exacerbated by excessive drinking, smoking, and other self-damaging behaviors. Conversely, in the case of suicide, anger is typically more prominent. Survivors struggle to reconcile themselves to the fact that suicide victims chose to die. Their anger is often linked to having been denied the opportunity to intervene with help. Fueling this anger is often a sense of helplessness. However, this acknowledgment of anger tends to be quickly followed by intense guilt, which effectively impedes the mourning process. Patients may go to great lengths to clarify and contradict previous descriptions of the lost person. They may emphatically deny that the situation was really as bad as they first described. Perhaps owing to displacement and projection, the guilt-ridden members often fear being "punished" by the other members.

Patients who express unpopular thoughts and feelings are in fact often reprimanded by those who are uncomfortable with acknowledging their own similar reactions. Comments such as "You should be relieved the jerk left you!" or "Don't be sad, there are many fish in the sea!" are typical and serve to counteract and neutralize a member's sorrow over a divorce. It seems to be easier to acknowledge anger at partners who have abandoned them than sadness over the loss and the fear of being alone. Apparently, it is dangerous for even one member to experience such affect. Perhaps they fear the contagion of such emotions. They may also fear overwhelming each other, thereby destroying the group. Tolerating the ambivalent feelings of anger, sadness, guilt, and relief is confusing, leading to a sense of being more conflicted about the loss and their feelings concerning the loss.

THE TERMINATION STAGE

The time limit is an integral part of addressing loss. Termination represents a unique opportunity for the patients to explore and reexperience their idiosyncratic reactions to loss that have created so much difficulty for them in the past. Therefore, each member's reaction to the loss of the group is interpreted as being a familiar pattern originating in the past. In addition, shared or group themes elicited by the termination are systematically explored. The inherent difficulties consequent of their patterns are identified. By understanding the relationship between their current feelings about termination and their past reactions to losses, patients can experiment with different and more adaptive reactions to loss. Hence the loss of the group can also serve as a rehearsal for future losses. We believe that the degree of ease with which patients accept ambivalent feelings about the therapist, the group members, the group experience, the end of the group, and the memory of past lost objects indicates the diminished impact of past (and future) losses. The loss groups offer patients the opportunity to understand and utilize their reactions to the loss of the group as a model for beginning to work through the unresolved conflicts associated with their previous losses.

As the termination stage begins, the therapist's repeated interpretations about the loss of the group begin to sink in. The theme of termination becomes focal. Conflicts associated with this theme include the hope for benefit versus the fear of repeated disappointment and abandonment. The danger of becoming close to each other echoes throughout the sessions. The patients reevaluate their commitment to the 12-week contract. The fear of facing more goodbyes may influence some patients' decision to drop out at this late point. Such departures offer the remainers a here-and-now opportunity to work through yet another experience of loss. Their reactions to the "late" dropouts can also be explored with respect to the extent to which they mirror reactions to past losses. The theme of survivor guilt may again predominate the group's reaction to the dropout.

Another theme that emerges prominently during the termination stage is that of change. Patients' conflicts related to this theme include the wish to live their lives differently versus the fear of changing their lives for the worse. In addition, there are fears of being incapable of changing and of taking the risks required to change. For example, to form new relationships demands that they be willing to be vulnerable. Defensively, they may cling to the past because it is familiar, albeit unsatisfying and even frustrating. Inevitably the patients begin to report that changes have been gradually occurring as they experiment with new behaviors outside the group as well as within the group. Ongoing relationships outside the group may become stressed when patients finally acknowledge their previously disavowed feelings. Many patients have tended to nurture others, for example, many adult children of alcoholics are involved in our loss groups. They experience much apprehension when they choose to confront their friends and family with issues they have long avoided. As they begin to experiment with changing these patterns of relating, they become frightened of the future and of the unknown. As they recognize the changes they are making, the theme of resolving the mourning begins to evolve.

Fears associated with resolving the mourning often result in fears of forgetting the other person ever existed. They fear their memories of the lost person will disappear with their grief. The therapist may interpret this fear of "throwing the baby out with the bathwater." The patients also express feeling incomplete without the lost person. However, they also express a sense of beginning to feel complete when alone. They also begin to recognize the various transitional objects that have come to represent the lost person. They may begin to consider putting away framed photographs of the lost one, taking off wedding bands, or donating the lost one's clothing to charity. Similarly, hobbies once shared with the lost one tend to become less interesting with time.

Within the group, members increasingly confront each other as they recognize in each other their own self-deceptions and false assumptions regarding death. It is also common for patients to begin the painful recognition of the reality of their own contribution to the losses. They struggle to accept the fact that they are the constant in a series of failed relationships. In this respect, some may consider the possibility of dating again. Ideally, they begin to choose partners that differ from those who have repeatedly disappointed them in the past. They struggle with their difficulties trusting again versus the loneliness of remaining solitary.

The next section presents the last session of the group. Many common themes elicited by the termination are represented. The session was attended by all its remaining members: Alice, Kyle, Michel, Margaret, Sarah, and Lois. The session began with Alice pointing out that she was sitting in a different seat, hiding from the one-way mirror. For the first time since the initial session, there was an animated discussion about the "secret observers" behind the one-way mirror, and the research staff. After several minutes the therapist intervened:

(001) THERAPIST: Well, you know, I guess what we're dealing with is the issue of trust. Can you really trust me to make sure that the people back there would be compassionate and understanding and professional enough not to mock the way you dress or not to chat to
(005) everybody on the street about the problems you're experiencing? So it's really a question of can you trust me to protect you from these secret observers.

MARGARET: But can we trust the results of the research? What will the results be?

(010) SARAH: That's interesting, eh? It would be interesting to know.

ALICE: Well, I feel great, I don't know why.

MARGARET: Because it's the last session.

SARAH: You're graduating. You must have felt great. When I was walking up I thought, who is the girl who is smiling away?

(015) ALICE: I like these sessions, though. I know I'll miss them. But maybe it is a relief in a way I don't even recognize yet. You know what I mean, like something is finished, I can go on with my life.

SARAH: I never thought of it that way.

THERAPIST: So the feeling is that you are going to miss the group and
(020)   each other and also feeling some relief. I wonder if there are any
other feelings with respect to the end of the group and saying
goodbye to each other and me.

MARGARET: I think I feel a little angry that I don't know what progress
I've made. I went to see my doctor yesterday as well, you know.
(025)   She says, "How are you doing?" and I said, "I don't know." I think
I'm doing fine, I have my ups and my downs, nothing's changed
there. Except I'm feeling better, I know, overall.

THERAPIST: So perhaps there are some feelings that—or some wishes,
anyway—that I would give you an evaluation, you know, your
(030)   graduation ceremony today; that I give you feedback or the research staff give you some feedback or judgment on how well
you've done or haven't done. So there seem to be some feelings
about my role, perhaps, and what I'm not giving you today.

LOIS: What bothers me is, I don't know whether I feel better as a result
(035)   of the medication or this group or because I've been reading a lot
of books I think have helped me—I don't know. But maybe it
doesn't really matter.

MICHEL: Well, I wonder why we can't have feedback.

THERAPIST: Well, it's a way of avoiding putting yourself in the driver's
(040)   seat and deciding for yourself how you feel regardless of what I
may think, or the people behind the mirror, or the research staff.
But I guess that might mean having to trust yourself.

MARGARET: I think I trust myself as long as things are going fine. But
if I have a setback, then I feel, oh my god.

(045) ALICE: That's when I start to feel scared too.

MARGARET: I still feel scared that I may have another loss or another
situation which will get me worked up and that I will quickly not
be able to handle it . . .

THERAPIST: Well, I guess you have a loss right here, the loss of each
(050)   other, which perhaps is not as profound a loss as the loss that
brought you into the group, but you are saying that you'll miss
each other.

MARGARET: I guess I made up my mind that if I had any losses in the
future I wouldn't deny that they were losses; that I would let
(055)   myself feel the loss. Now whether I do it with the loss of this
group, maybe I won't because I tend to feel that I'm not going to
let the loss of this group bother me and maybe I feel that it
shouldn't bother me.

SARAH: I felt sad last night. I was thinking about the fact I had to come
(060)   today and I felt quite sad that maybe it was too soon to end it for
          me and for others and that it was too bad it was set up that way,
          but—

MARGARET: I was reading the paper and it was a very sad story and
          tears came to my eyes. And I was going to stop the feeling right
(065)   then and there but I thought no, I will feel sad because it was sad,
          and I can cry a few tears if I'm sad. So maybe that's a realization
          that I do shut things off immediately.

There is a discussion about the "silly" things that make them cry. They
also discuss people they know who cry "over nothing."

(070) THERAPIST: Well, you know, we're hearing about people out there, and
          earlier we were hearing about wanting judgments and feedback.
          I guess what we're not hearing about is how you feel about each
          other in here. And maybe the fear is that you'll be judged nega-
          tively in here, that people will think you're overly emotional for
(075)   feeling that you'll miss each other in here. In any case, there seems
          to be an avoidance of directly giving feedback in here to each
          other.

MARGARET: Well, we could do that.

ALICE: Kyle, you start.

(080) KYLE: Thanks!

SARAH: I think Kyle is a lot more relaxed.

KYLE: I do feel a lot better than when I first came in. Like I say, there
          are days too when I'm just putting on a big act. I feel all tied up
          inside. But I'm starting to relax and not get so keyed up about
(085)   things. Like the song says, "We don't need another hero."

SARAH: Well, I feel in this group that I have learned a lot about myself;
          that my feelings count. And you know, just to have someone sit
          here and listen to what I have to say and not think I'm, you know,
          off the wall or something like that is a real relief to me. I had my
(090)   mother all those years to sit there and sort of set me straight on
          things and then when she died, I was sort of on my own, and I
          started doubting the way I was feeling about things. Within the
          last twelve weeks, I go three times a week to exercise classes at
          lunch time during work now, I'm taking riding lessons, something
(095)   I've wanted to do my whole life, and I'm playing ball again once
          a week. Things that I didn't do because I figured my responsibility
          is to everybody else, not myself. (Sarah continues by discussing

all she used to do for her husband and children and how some of their personal habits "drive me crazy.")

(100) THERAPIST: And maybe that's the fear in here: that to give feedback means you'd have to mention each other's personal habits that "drive you crazy."

ALICE: Well, I could pass my opinion of what I thought, but I wouldn't want to leave here with hard feelings, you know. Like I could say
(105) how I felt, maybe just skim the surface for each person, but that would be all. I couldn't say exactly what I thought, because I don't really know the whole person. I think it would be unfair of me to pass a judgment because I don't really know all of you really well.

THERAPIST: So you're protecting each other from fear that you'd hurt
(110) their feelings or there would be bad feelings.

MARGARET: Well, that's a point, because I think we do rescue. I rescue my husband and my son, and bosses: I always feel I need to rescue men. I guess because I never rescued my father.

ALICE: I have to be honest. I think you're [*Looking at Michel*] too quiet.
(115) I think you could have added more to the sessions but maybe that is your character. I might be wrong, I don't know, but I feel like you could have contributed more. That's being honest. As a person you seem like a nice, quiet, soft-spoken person that way, but—

MARGARET: No, I'm worried. Michel causes me to worry and I get mad
(120) at him because I'm worrying about him because I think he is very depressed.

MICHEL: No, I'm quiet in here but during the week I'm going all the time.

MARGARET: Yeah, but I think you're depressed when you're going all
(125) the time. That's the feeling you've given me anyway.

MICHEL: Well, the thing is I understand my wife and I sympathize with her. She married when she was 21 but she never had any fun. She was restricted to just the house, she couldn't go out with her friends. She couldn't go to the bar, she couldn't join anything,
(130) things like that. And then it hit her. Like it's her life and she's missed out and so she goes for it but where am I? I'm just left behind.

ALICE: That's what I went through too.

MICHEL: Yeah, I know. You make me think of my wife, and I understand
(135) her now. But it doesn't help. I'm still left behind.

LOIS: I know how you feel. It was hard for me to accept that my marriage was over. I was very nervous starting to date again. I just felt, What's the point? I didn't want to start over again, I wanted my husband back. I'd look for him everywhere. The first time I (140)   went to a dance at the singles' club, I kept looking for him.

The other members share similar experiences about lost loves and starting over.

THERAPIST: I think what the group is saying to Michel is that by hanging on to your wife and hoping that she'll come back, you (145)   stop yourself from really getting involved with new people. Even in here, not really wanting to admit that your wife is gone and it has prevented you from getting involved in here.

MARGARET: Well, I want some feedback from you too. I think I've been the saddest one here because I have cried the most, I think. So what (150)   do I look like to you? Someone who is really unstable and cries too much?

KYLE: You cried for all of us.

The group gives Margaret some very pointed yet supportive feedback concerning her difficulties and her role in the group.

(155) MARGARET: I think I've gotten a lot out of the group and I worry because I don't think Michel has. I think maybe I've taken too much of the group's time.

ALICE: I don't agree with that. I think we're all given the opportunity. We either have the courage to speak up and talk or we don't. I (160)   think that it is just a matter of, you know, if you decide to be silent, well then you can't expect people to help you or to know you.

KYLE: I made the decision to sit and nod my head wisely. But then I thought: Am I going to help myself or not?

MARGARET: Well, I know I can't take on all your worries.

(165) ALICE: No.

MARGARET: You mentioned last week that you'd like to do housework for me and I thought it was a good idea and then I thought, it's not a good idea because—

ALICE: No, it isn't, I know.

(170) MARGARET: Because I know too much of your problems and I'm sure I'd want to know how you are doing.

ALICE: I thought about it too and I thought I'll want to know if you're doing well.

MARGARET: We know too much about each other from here.

(175) ALICE: I've applied for several other jobs. I think that's best.

MARGARET: I guess I don't want another daughter after all.

ALICE: And like she (the therapist) said it's a way of not letting go of the group. Oh look, I'm crying.

The members ask Alice about the different jobs for which she has (180) applied, whether she has obtained interviews, and so forth.

THERAPIST: Maybe that's one of the hardest things about saying good-bye: You won't know how the stories turn out; what could've been; what might've been.

SARAH: Well, I want to know what's going to happen to Michel. I think (185) I protect him, uh you, because I was feeling like your wife. I was scared my marriage would break up if I started doing things for myself.

THERAPIST: I guess you feel guilty when you're doing things for yourself and that's very unusual for all of you, to put yourself as a (190) priority, and I'm wondering about in here, if there are some feelings of guilt about the fact that you may have gotten more out of the group than other people. And if you want to fix it by rescuing Michel before the clock ticks away on this last session.

SARAH: For me it started with my mom's death. I guess maybe just (195) thinking about my own mortality and what have I done? What have I done with my life? Like you know, I haven't. I have no education, I wanted to go back to school. I've been working since I was 15. God, this is my life! My mom worked all her life, and for what?

(200) MARGARET: I admire the fact that you have chosen to take some time for yourself and I want to follow your example. I want to take two and a half hours during the week to do something for myself 'cause it takes two and a half hours to come to this group if you count travel time. But I can't decide what to do.

(205) There is a discussion about what Margaret can do.

MARGARET: I put it down as one of my goals: to get into a health fitness routine because I need to lose weight and exercise more. Didn't

everyone put down goals for therapy? Above that I put something
about trying to find out why I need to control others, because I do
(210)   like to control others. I like to control my children, I like to control
my boss, I'd like to control the government of Canada.

There is a joyful discussion about the government of Canada and how
incompetent its leader is.

THERAPIST: I guess Margaret was bringing up the idea of wanting
(215)   self-control and that wanting to control others is in some ways a
response to feeling helpless and out of control and how frightening that is.

MARGARET: I think that's what I learned and I'd never thought of that.
I want to control my children because I know best. But the fact is
(220)   that I do at times feel very helpless. And so if I'm feeling helpless
it's much easier for me to tell my husband what he should do or
tell my daughter how she should clean up her act than for me to
clean up my act.

SARAH: Yeah.

(225) THERAPIST: I think the helplessness is another emotion that you feel in
response to the loss. Feeling that you have no control over the loss,
that you're feeling helpless, and again with this group you have
no control over the fact this group is going to end today and
perhaps there is a sense of helplessness there too. And I also would
(230)   imagine your helplessness would make you feel angry with me
for ending the group today.

MARGARET: I don't feel angry at you. I feel angry against the University
of Alberta psychiatric unit that sets up these research projects and
sets up a group like this, because I guess I want to know what's
(235)   next and that's why I went to my doctor yesterday—because I was
feeling I have to have a plan after this or I won't know what to do.
So I've got to have a safety net.

SARAH: Yeah.

THERAPIST: I'm struck by how in some ways, Margaret, your pattern
(240)   continues with the loss of this group. Your wish is to replace this
with something else before the group even ends. You want to
avoid the sadness or any of the feelings associated with saying
goodbye by having your safety net; something to replace this
group with.

(245) MARGARET: That has been a pattern, I know. I knew when I was
carrying my last baby the child was encephalic and wouldn't live,

so we made plans that we would adopt right afterwards, which we did.

LOIS: So it's a real pattern for you; an avoidance of feeling alone.

(250) MARGARET: But that to me is just like good planning; I don't want to be alone. [*Pause*] And yet I'm not alone, so why do I feel that way? I have so many people around.

MICHEL: Well, you could be with a whole bunch of people and still feel alone, because it's, oh, how can I say this? I guess you don't get (255) the response that you need for yourself or something like that, not necessarily the affection.

MARGARET: But I guess that's also the thing that stops me too when I say I don't want another daughter. I don't even want another friend because with friendships, with the good things comes the (260) loss [*Crying*] and I've done that before where I've met someone and I've thought I really like them; we should become friends. And maybe they've even made overtures to me and I don't make them back because I know I have friends scattered right across the country who write to me and they phone me and I'm never the (265) one to initiate any, very seldom to initiate any contact with them.

ALICE: I know what you mean. I used to think that something was so terribly wrong with me, I would feel so depressed and so sad. All I want in my life is to be happy, so why can't I be happy? And like I was saying before, it was like I would always—even if I was (270) happy—I'd be looking for something that was going to make me sad and I don't know why. I'm still like that. But I guess just since I came to this group and since I've decided to do something about it, I guess I just sort of made up my mind that, well, you know, if I'm the only one that's preventing myself from being happy, I'm (275) going to have to change my thinking around.

Margaret talks about her family and the theme of loneliness.

THERAPIST: I don't think it's surprising that these things are coming up as you're saying goodbye to each other today and you're faced again with another loss: the loss of the group. And one of the (280) feelings that is really triggering all of you is this fear of being alone, of being sad and giving up; of lying down and dying.

MARGARET: I was never afraid of dying because I think it would be very nice and peaceful if one could choose how one dies. You just go to sleep and die and never have to wake up.

(285) SARAH: I thought a lot about dying when my mom died. I must admit that it really bothered me.

ALICE: I was watching Pollyanna . . . [*Describes a scene from the movie*] . . . You know, how can you contemplate death when you're alive? You have to—well, you can but you shouldn't be looking—It's like
(290)   looking on the bad side of something before it happens, you know? Instead of saying okay, I have my whole life ahead of me. Look at it that way. If something happens, that's fine. But right now you're alive.

MARGARET: I've been a Pollyanna all my life. Like I know this group is
(295)   ending and I'm just telling myself I'm not going to be sad about it; I'm going to be glad I had the experience; be glad for the good that I got out of it. Yet I'm denying how I'm really feeling about the group. But I still think you have to imagine the good things, even if you're only fooling yourself in order to carry on. I'm
(300)   reading a book about healing yourself through imagery. . . .

MICHEL: Is it okay to talk about Ellen?

SARAH: Hm, I wonder how she's doing.

MARGARET: I hope she got some help.

KYLE: Wouldn't it be funny if she showed up to say goodbye.

(305) [*Laughter*]

MICHEL: While we're talking about the group, do you [*To therapist*] mind answering a question? What was the data you were trying to get from the group? Do you understand what I'm getting at? Let's say we're like the group here and one day you say to Alice,
(310)   stay home and see how the rest of the group is going to react. Since we don't get more input from you, or you don't give us what to do or what to say or how to behave, then you study—were you studying the situation?

Other group members intervened at this point, attempting to answer
(315) Michel's question.

SARAH: I know what Michel's saying: When one of us doesn't show up, you always want to know how we feel about that person not sitting in the chair. Because this is a loss group and we're supposed to concentrate on loss, and when someone isn't here we should
(320)   recognize how little or how small it is in the measurement of loss in the past. It's a loss and we should discuss that loss because maybe we could understand our other losses if we understand how we handle this loss.

MICHEL: Yeah, how we behave in different situations that are arising
(325)   from our losses or something like that. Like the first lady that was
          here and you asked us if it bothered us because she didn't come
          back. It did bother us the first day, but after that, well—because
          we didn't know her really. She was just like part of the furniture.
          She didn't, you know, communicate or things like that. I just don't
(330)   understand what exactly, what it was all about, you know, as far
          as I'm concerned I didn't get much out of it. I mean I understand
          a lot of things, like, whatever you are talking about and thinking,
          and I sympathize with everyone here.

MARGARET: But you didn't personally get much for yourself.

(335) MICHEL: No, not what I needed.

THERAPIST: And I guess that is very similar to your marriage where
          you, after it was over, still didn't know what it was all about except
          that your needs were not met and you felt left behind.

MICHEL: No, I understand my marriage. But I don't know what I need.

(340) ALICE: Yeah, I was going to say, What do you need?

MICHEL: That's it. I don't know what I need right now and this is why
          I came to this group.

LOIS: You sound panicked. But Michel, you hardly ever talked. You
          only get out what you put in, you know. It's like you thought if
(345)   you just showed up here, things would change.

THERAPIST: I guess I'm hearing some disappointment about what you
          didn't get out of the group. And I don't think Michel is the only
          one who feels somewhat disappointed. Margaret was sort of
          hinting at that earlier. But I guess it's hard to talk about that.

(350) MICHEL: Yeah, nothing's solved. I'm still alone.

ALICE: You do sound disappointed.

MICHEL: No, it's okay. Whatever I got, what little bit I got out of it, you
          know, I'll just go from there and join another therapy or whatever.

MARGARET: I expected a lot and I'm disappointed, because I would like
(355)   to have my expectations met. I think maybe I'm going to need
          more and I didn't want to have to need something more. I wanted
          to come to this group and get better and never be sick again. I
          guess I have to learn to feel sadness when it's there and not say it
          doesn't matter and also feel happiness. I was shrugging those off
(360)   too because it's going to be a long struggle for the rest of my life.
          But at least I think now that I have accepted that I was depressed.
          I mean it sounds silly to say that but, like my sister, she used to

say, "Mustn't be depressed: that's very dangerous for our family;
you have to fight against being depressed." And that's what I have
(365)   been trying to do all my life. But that book I was talking about.
Now that was really helpful.

THERAPIST: I think this might be another way of saying to me that what
this group didn't give you, you'll have to get elsewhere, whether
in other therapies or books. Sort of telling me what you didn't get
(370)   from me. I think it's been very difficult for you to express how you
feel about me, as if I have no impact on you at all. I wonder what
it is you do feel, if it's anger, disappointment. Since I didn't give
you what you wanted from me, it's as if I have given you nothing,
and I'm not even here.

(375) MICHEL: I don't think we're angry. I think we understand that it's your
job and that's it, that's all.

ALICE: Noncommittal type.

MICHEL: Well, your job, not to really get involved or care.

ALICE: You advise when you should advise. I don't feel angry with you
(380)   at all. I think I will miss you. I don't know why, maybe just because
you're always here, you're the silent mother.

MARGARET: Well, you have made statements that have helped me. I felt
that when I say something and you respond, whether you're
responding to me or whether you're responding to someone else,
(385)   I've understood what you're trying to get at. At least I have more
in the later part. In the first part I didn't know.

ALICE: No, me either.

LOIS: I guess I was feeling angry when you kept referring to Ellen
because I thought—

(390) MARGARET: [Interrupting] How can you miss her when you don't even
know her? Yeah, I can't lose something I never had.

KYLE: But then again, Margaret, you missed your children and you
never knew them either.

MARGARET: Oh! [Pause] my, [Pause] that's true.

(395) SARAH: Well, I just didn't understand a lot of what you were saying at
the beginning until a couple of sessions past. I went home and was
telling George, well, maybe she was trying to get you to talk more
about why you're there, your loss, you know. Whereas I came in
and I didn't want to talk about it at all, you know.

(400) THERAPIST: And you also didn't want to feel anything for Ellen, and

you didn't want to feel anything for each other, or for anybody ever again, because it hurts.

ALICE: But I remember that first session with her.

SARAH: Yeah, when everybody was so silent!

(405) ALICE: And she made me feel so upset and sad inside.

MARGARET: We might have had a better group if Ellen had come. Maybe we should be mad at her for not coming. She could have helped us.

ALICE: Well, I found it quite disturbing that she was so quiet and she
(410) was so sad.

SARAH: She started talking a bit, remember. And then we started talking about our anxiety attacks. She just got really shook up and started crying and she wouldn't even look up after awhile. I felt really sorry for her. I mean we didn't know why she was crying
(415) because she wouldn't say, you know; when you asked her, she wouldn't talk.

ALICE: Actually, I'm glad that I attended these sessions. One reason is that my sister, Mary, you know I couldn't—my friends couldn't relate to the fact that I felt a loss or that I grieved over the loss of
(420) my sister fifteen years ago. It's like my close friends, they never lost a mother or their father yet. They haven't lost brothers or sisters, you know, or if they have they don't ever show it. They don't talk about it, so it's like "Why, Alice, that was fifteen years ago."

(425) MARGARET: Yeah, "Get over it, smarten up."

ALICE: And so instead, I kept it inside, and then in here, with you people that maybe don't understand everything, but do understand, or are trying to understand the different feelings. I feel like I can unload and you people will try to understand, even if you
(430) don't.

SARAH: You don't know everything about me, so it's like an objective opinion. It's like I'm not going to lose anything by telling you.

LOIS: Safe.

MARGARET: Yeah, it was safe to cry in here.

(435) THERAPIST: Well, I guess it's time for us to say goodbye.

MARGARET: Yeah, I noticed it was 11:30.

ALICE: Is it really?

SARAH: Kyle hardly spoke at all.

KYLE: Goodbye. [*Other members exchange goodbyes.*]

This twelfth and final session of the group elicited many of the aforementioned themes that characterize the termination stage. Two themes were particularly focal. They were "judgement day" and "goodbye." The opening discussion of the "secret observers" was perhaps inaccurately interpreted by the therapist (001-007) as reflecting the theme of trust. The theme was, however, clarified by Margaret as involving judgment day: "But can we trust the results of the research? What will the results be?" (008-009). Although the therapist's intervention might have missed the mark, it is instructive to note the unfolding of the patients' response to the therapist. Unlike earlier sessions where the therapist's interventions seemed to be ignored, even when they seemed accurate, at this point her interpretation elicited a clarifying response. The segment that followed reflected several aspects of the judgment day theme. A primary aspect was the source of the evaluation. On the one hand, Alice immediately took the initiative and offered an evaluation of her own progress and her feelings regarding ending the group:

ALICE: Well, I feel great . . . I like these sessions, though. I know I'll miss them. But maybe it is a relief in a way I don't even recognize yet. You know what I mean, like something is finished, I can go on with my life. (011-017)

Margaret, however, countered this self-evaluation by introducing her doctor as a hoped-for source of evaluation:

MARGARET: I think I feel a little angry that I don't know what progress I've made. I went to see my doctor yesterday as well, you know. She says, "How are you doing?" and I said, "I don't know." I think I'm doing fine, I have my ups and my downs, nothing's changed there. Except I'm feeling better, I know, overall. (023-027)

Lois's comment reflected that she had joined Alice's camp in that she could accept the ambiguity of evaluating her progress:

LOIS: What bothers me, is I don't know whether I feel better as a result of the medication or this group or because I've been reading a lot of books I think have helped me—I don't know. *But maybe it doesn't really matter.* (034-037)

Michel, however, persisted with the wish for the therapist to evaluate him: "Well, I wonder why we can't have feedback" (038). At that point the therapist interpreted the defense against autonomy, mastery, and self-evaluation:

THERAPIST: Well, it's a way of avoiding putting yourself in the driver's seat and deciding for yourself how you feel regardless of what I may think, or the people behind the mirror, or the research staff. But I guess that might mean having to trust yourself. (039-042)

Margaret's response clarified the fear behind the defense as being her fear of the future: "I think I trust myself as long as things are going fine. But if I have a setback, then I feel, oh my god." (043-044).

The therapist later attempted to provide the group with the opportunity for appraising their progress by focusing on the painful here-and-now situation of the loss of the group:

THERAPIST: Well, I guess you have a loss right here, the loss of each other, which perhaps is not as profound a loss as the loss that brought you into the group, but you are saying that you'll miss each other. (049-052)

In this way the theme of judgment became linked with the theme of saying goodbye. We believe that the manner in which the patients address the end of the group reflects how much they have learned about coping with loss. The therapist's goal with respect to termination is to foster the experience and expression of the many emotions associated with loss. We believe that by tolerating their ambivalence with respect to the loss of the group and of each other, the patients will be better equipped to face subsequent losses in their lives.

The patients responded to the therapist's implicit invitation by beginning to evaluate their progress in dealing with the loss at hand, that is, the loss of the group. Margaret struggled with the significance of the loss:

MARGARET: I guess I made up my mind that if I had any losses in the future I wouldn't deny that they were losses; that I would let myself feel the loss. Now whether I do it with the loss of this group, maybe I won't because I tend to feel that I'm not going to let the loss of this group bother me and *maybe I feel that it shouldn't bother me.* (053-058)

Conversely, we believe that Sarah's statement reflected her acceptance of the significance of the loss of the group, her acknowledgment of her disappointment regarding its loss, and her acceptance of her disappointment.

SARAH: I felt sad last night. I was thinking about the fact I had to come today and I felt quite sad that maybe it was too soon to end it for me and for others and that it was too bad it was set up that way, but— (059-062)

The fear behind the patients' reluctance to address the here-and-now loss became clear and was interpreted by the therapist: "And maybe the fear is that you'll be judged negatively in here, that people will think you're overly emotional for feeling that you'll miss each other in here" (073-075). With the therapist's implicit encouragement, they attempted to evaluate their progress by themselves, starting with the reluctant Kyle:

KYLE: I do feel a lot better than when I first came in. Like I say, there are days too when I'm just putting on a big act. I feel all tied up inside. But I'm starting to relax and not get so keyed up about things. Like the song says, "We don't need another hero." (082-085)

Sarah continued this self-evaluation but avoided extending this evaluation to the other members: "Well, I feel in this group that I have learned a lot about myself; that my feelings count. . . ." (086-087). The fear behind the avoidance of giving direct feedback to each other was elaborated by Alice:

ALICE: Well, I could pass my opinion of what I thought, but I *wouldn't want to leave here with hard feelings,* you know. Like I could say how I felt, maybe just skim the surface for each person, but that would be all. I couldn't say exactly what I thought, because I don't really know the whole person. I think it would be unfair of me to pass a judgment because I don't really know all of you really well. (103-108)

The defense and the fear were interpreted by the therapist: "So you're protecting each other from fear that you'd hurt their feelings or there would be bad feelings" (109-110). Alice took the initiative again and apprehensively confronted Michel:

ALICE: I have to be honest. I think you're too quiet. I think you could have added more to the sessions but maybe that is your character.

I might be wrong, I don't know, but I feel like you could have contributed more. That's being honest. As a person you seem like a nice, quiet, soft-spoken person that way, but— (114-118)

Her confrontation was supported by Margaret: "No, I'm worried. Michel causes me to worry and I get mad at him because I'm worrying about him because I think he is very depressed" (119-121).

Although Michel initially dismissed their concern (122-123), he finally did respond by describing his dilemma concerning his divorce (126-132). The group responded to his dilemma by empathizing with his difficulties (133-140). The therapist also addressed the dynamics underlying these difficulties (143-147). At that point Margaret diverted the group's attention away from Michel. In a sense she rescued Michel by inviting the members to criticize or praise her: "So what do I look like to you? Someone who is really unstable and who cries too much?" (149-151). Whereas Margaret tended to fulfill the role of the Professional Nurturer in the group, Kyle astutely identified her other role as the Emotional Conductor: "You cried for all of us" (152). Margaret attempted to return the floor to Michel but Alice preempted, colluding with Michel's dependency:

ALICE: I don't agree with that. I think we're all given the opportunity. We either have the courage to speak up and talk or we don't. I think that it is just a matter of, you know, if you decide to be silent, well then you can't expect people to help you or to know you. (158-161)

While Michel maintained his role as the Monk, Kyle responded non-defensively: "I made the decision to sit and nod my head wisely. But then I thought: Am I going to help myself or not?" (162-163). Margaret next explored her role as the Professional Nurturer, deciding "I don't want another daughter, after all" (176). At that point Sarah again attempted to return the focus to Michel: "I want to know what's going to happen to Michel . . . " (184). However, it seemed that Michel was still too hot to handle, and several themes evolved before the focus finally returned to him.

One theme that evolved during this middle segment involved survivor guilt versus doing something good for yourself and enjoying life:

SARAH: For me it started with my mom's death. I guess maybe just thinking about my own mortality and what have I done? (194-195)

MARGARET: I admire the fact that you have chosen to take some time for yourself and I want to follow your example. (200-201)

ALICE: I would feel so depressed and so sad. . . . I'd be looking for something that was going to make me sad and I don't know why. . . . if I'm the only one that's preventing myself from being happy, I'm going to have to change my thinking around. (267-275)

The theme of helplessness also evolved, which the therapist linked to the loss of the group:

THERAPIST: I think the helplessness is another emotion that you feel in response to the loss. Feeling that you have no control over the loss, that you're feeling helpless, and again with this group you have no control over the fact this group is going to end today and perhaps there is a sense of helplessness there too. And I also would imagine your helplessness would make you feel angry with me for ending the group today. (225-231)

The theme of helplessness evolved into the theme of loneliness and loss, which the therapist again linked to the termination:

THERAPIST: I don't think it's surprising that these things are coming up as you're saying goodbye to each other today and you're faced again with another loss: the loss of the group. And one of the feelings that is really triggering all of you is this fear of being alone, of being sad and giving up; of *lying down and dying*. (277-281)

As reviewed in Chapter 2, the association between being alone and dying is consistent with the dependency of this population. As previously mentioned, the theme of mortality commonly emerges in the loss groups around the midway mark. The theme of one's own mortality, however, tends to emerge only fleetingly. It rarely develops into a focal theme. In this session a few members responded to the therapist's identification of this existential theme.

MARGARET: I was never afraid of dying because I think it would be very nice and peaceful if one could choose how one dies. You just go to sleep and die and never have to wake up.

SARAH: I thought a lot about dying when my mom died. I must admit that it really bothered me.

ALICE: You know, how can you contemplate death when you're alive? You have to—well, you can but you shouldn't be looking—It's like looking on the bad side of something before it happens, you know? Instead of saying okay, I have my whole life ahead of me. Look at it that way. If something happens, that's fine. But right now you're alive. (282-293)

At that point Michel brought up this group's "dead" by asking if he could talk about Ellen (301). With his question the focus had finally returned to Michel (306).

Michel confronted the therapist, asking for a rationale for the way in which she had conducted the group. Initially he only hinted at his dissatisfaction: "Since we don't get more input from you, or you don't give us what to do or what to say or how to behave . . . " (310-312). Later he rejected Sarah's rationale (316-323) for focusing on the "empty chair," and his dissatisfaction was becoming more obvious:

MICHEL: . . . because we didn't know her really. She was just like part of the furniture. She didn't, you know, communicate or things like that. I just don't understand what exactly, what it was all about, you know, as far as I'm concerned I didn't get much out of it. (327-331)

His rejection of the importance of Ellen is noteworthy, given the fact that he had earlier raised her from the dead: "Is it okay to talk about Ellen?" (301). The therapist attempted to link Michel's current feeling regarding the loss of the group with the loss of his marriage:

THERAPIST: And I guess that is very similar to your marriage where you, after it was over, still didn't know what it was all about except that your needs were not met and you felt left behind. (336-338)

He rejected her interpretation but did clarify his concern: "No, I understand my marriage. But I don't know what I need." (339) Lois's statement to Michel suggested that he was in danger of being scapegoated:

LOIS: But Michel, you hardly ever talked. You only get out what you put in, you know. It's like you thought if you just showed up here things would change. (343-345)

The therapist's intervention addressed Michel's disappointment as fulfilling a role for the group:

THERAPIST: I guess I'm hearing some disappointment about what you didn't get out of the group. And I don't think Michel is the only one who feels somewhat disappointed. Margaret was sort of hinting at that earlier. But I guess it's hard to talk about that. (346-349)

As with any group therapy experience, there is variability in the gains achieved by the patients. Michel was clearly acknowledging that he was not satisfied. In response, the others could have attempted to quiet his doubts and convince him that the group was beneficial to him. Instead the group tried to cure him. Failing this, the group seemed to be gearing up to scapegoat this "doubting Thomas." Margaret responded to the therapist's interpretation of Michel's role by acknowledging her disappointment: "I expected a lot and I'm disappointed because I would like to have my expectations met . . . " (354-355). The therapist focused the disappointment on herself:

THERAPIST: I think this might be another way of saying to me that what this group didn't give you, you'll have to get elsewhere, whether in other therapies or books. Sort of telling me what you didn't get from me. (367-370)

This interpretation reflected the belief that the anger that was directed at Michel may have been displaced from the therapist onto him. It was unlikely that Michel remained the only member who had doubts about the therapist's contribution. Such doubts would be consistent with the anger and disappointment felt toward former frustrating objects. Conversely, the friction among the members may also have served the purpose of reducing the pain and sadness of the goodbye by diminishing the significance of the loss.

Although the therapist's interpretation was overtly denied, the disappointment with her was nevertheless clear:

MICHEL: I don't think we're angry. I think we understand that it's your job and that's it, that's all.

ALICE: Noncommittal type.

MICHEL: Well, your job, not to really get involved or care. (375-378)

The section that followed (379-399) involved somewhat of an evaluation of the therapist. It was balanced in that they conveyed their appreciation as well as their frustration:

ALICE: You advise when you should advise. I don't feel angry with you at all. I think I will miss you. I don't know why, maybe just because you're always here, *you're the silent mother.*

MARGARET: Well, you have made statements that have helped me. . . . I've understood what you're trying to get at. At least I have more in the later part. *In the first part I didn't know.*

ALICE: No, me either.

LOIS: I guess *I was feeling angry* when you kept referring to Ellen because I thought—

MARGARET: [*Interrupting*] How can you miss her when you don't even know her? *Yeah, I can't lose something I never had. . . .*

SARAH: Well, I just didn't understand a lot of what you were saying at the beginning . . . I came in and I didn't want to talk about it at all, you know.

In the final segment of the session (403-439), the patients discussed their concern about the dropout and their appreciation of the group experience. This juxtaposition of the two themes suggested that they were comfortable with the fact that they were survivors. The guilt that had characterized previous discussions of Ellen was replaced by a more realistic appraisal (405-416) of her behavior in the group:

ALICE: And she made me feel so upset and sad inside.

MARGARET: We might have had a better group if Ellen had come. Maybe we should be mad at her for not coming. She could have helped us.

ALICE: Well, I found it quite disturbing that she was so quiet and she was so sad.

SARAH: She started talking a bit, remember. And then we started talking about our anxiety attacks. She just got really shook up and started crying and she wouldn't even look up after awhile. I felt really sorry for her. I mean we didn't know why she was crying because she wouldn't say, you know; when you asked her, she wouldn't talk.

To summarize this final session, a focal theme was that of the judgment day. A primary aspect of that theme was the source of the evaluation. Some wished that the therapist would praise them, offer feedback and evaluations; they were disappointed that such feedback was not forthcoming. Others reacted to this disappointment by evaluating themselves. They rewarded themselves for their accomplishments and felt empowered to alter their future. They disclosed that they had been practicing new assertiveness skills. They were increasingly tuning into their feelings and were pleased by the results. Contrary to their fears, they had not been deserted by friends and family. Rather, they reported feeling supported and encouraged, which tended to further heighten their sense of autonomy and mastery, and, hence, self-esteem.

In evaluating their progress, the patients were simultaneously evaluating the efficacy of their STG treatment. Throughout the session, they specifically identified factors that they found beneficial:

SARAH: Well, I feel in this group that I have learned a lot about myself; that my feelings count. And you know, just to have someone sit here and listen to what I have to say and not think I'm, you know, off the wall or something like that is a real relief to me. (086-089)

ALICE: I think we're all given the opportunity. We either have the courage to speak up and talk or we don't. I think that it is just a matter of, you know, if you decide to be silent, well then you can't expect people to help you or to know you. (158-161)

SARAH: Because this is a loss group and we're supposed to concentrate on loss, and when someone isn't here we should recognize how little or how small it is in the measurement of loss in the past. It's a loss and we should discuss that loss because maybe we could understand our other losses if we understand how we handle this loss. (318-323)

MARGARET: Well, you have made statements that have helped me. I felt that when I say something and you respond, whether you're responding to me or whether you're responding to someone else, I've understood what you're trying to get at. (382-385)

ALICE: In here, with you people that maybe don't understand everything, but do understand, or are trying to understand the different feelings. I feel like I can unload and you people will try to understand, even if you don't. (426-430)

SARAH: You don't know everything about me, so it's like an objective opinion. It's like I'm not going to lose anything by telling you. (431-432)

LOIS: Safe. (433)

MARGARET: Yeah, it was safe to cry in here. (434)

The other major theme that characterized this final session was that of saying goodbye. The goodbyes to the group as a whole and to the various individuals varied in their completeness. This variability perhaps suggested the level of work accomplished by individual patients. The many conflicts associated with this theme were also elicited.

Some conflicts were common to all members. For example, they wished to give the group a proper send-off: to have a wake or a graduation ceremony. At the same time, they feared the emotions associated with the group's funeral, avoiding the issue for some time. Some conflicts reflected individual dynamics. For example, a goal for Margaret seemed to be to tell Alice how close she felt to her. This disclosure may have helped her overcome regrets about things not said to a lost one. Their discussion was in sharp contrast to the one of the previous week wherein Alice had planned to do housecleaning for Margaret (166-178). That earlier conversation seemed to reflect the persistent fantasy that they could talk and share forever. Such a fantasy overlooked the need to say goodbye, the contribution of the safe confines of the therapy group, and the contribution of the therapist.

With reluctance the members began to say goodbye to the group. Their awareness that the group had not been perfect served to remind them that nothing is perfect or forever. They struggled to accept this painful reality. Part of this struggle was displayed in their evaluation of the therapist. They cautiously conveyed their ambivalence. By accepting their ambivalence, we believe that they are better armed to confront the loss of ambivalently held objects in the future.

SUMMARY

In this chapter we have presented the evolution of a loss group from its beginning stage through its termination session. We believe that the clinical material was an accurate demonstration of the richness of the processes that occur in our loss groups. The vignettes reflected common themes that have emerged in each STG we have conducted. By theme we refer to the specific content of a conflict that exists in the group over a period of time. Two types of group themes were represented by the clinical material: those that recurred throughout the life of the group and those that emerged in association with specific events or stages of the group.

The patients' behavior was also conceptualized as the formation of patient roles. By role we refer to a well-defined set of behaviors presented by a patient that represents a conflict shared by other patients. Although the behaviors (and conflict) may have appeared to belong only to the patient occupying the role, the role actually served a function for the entire group. Furthermore, each role served both a defensive and an adaptive function. Some emerged to fulfill what was wished for from the therapist; others emerged to fulfill other needs of the group. We identified six patient roles: the Apparition, the Monk, the Professional Nurturer, the Professor, the Emotional Conductor, and the Cruise Director.

The therapist was confronted by many challenges when conducting this loss group. We believe that some challenges reflected the nature of the patient population and others reflected the structure of the groups. The therapeutic techniques utilized to address the challenges and processes of STG were illustrated throughout the clinical vignettes. Our discussion emphasized two foci of therapist interpretations that we believe are central to the therapist technique. Those foci involved the interpretation of transference phenomena and of patients' reactions to an absent member. Our discussion of the therapist's interventions also represented our guidelines for addressing the challenges confronted by the STG therapist.

The vignettes depicted several factors that we believe facilitated the efficacy of STG. Those factors included the time limit; the group modality; the group's homogeneous composition, the therapist's focus on here-and-now interpersonal interactions and the linking of the same with past relationships; especially the lost relationship; and the exploration of member–member and member–therapist transference phenomena. As researchers we were interested in empirically evaluating the extent to which patients had indeed benefited from the group. We present the findings of the outcome study in Chapter 8. Let us first review, in Chapter 7, the literature on previous research evaluating the efficacy of group interventions for loss.

CHAPTER 7

Research Evaluations
of Group Interventions

Given the nature and magnitude of the problems associated with loss and the variety of available group intervention methods, one might assume that a number of studies have been conducted on the efficacy of group intervention methods for persons who have suffered a person loss. That does not appear to be the case. After reviewing the research literature, Shackelton (1984) stated:

> The first of two main conclusions from the summary of outcome studies is that their paucity contrasts with both the extent of theoretical writing and with the confidence with which treatments are recommended. The second is that serious methodological flaws mean the need remains for well-designed group outcome studies (for both clinical and research purposes). (p. 197)

Other reviewers (Raphael & Middleton, 1987; Stroebe & Stroebe, 1987) concur.

Our own review of the research literature revealed only five systematic studies of group intervention, all of which were published between 1978 and 1988 (Barrett, 1978; Lieberman & Videka-Sherman, 1986; Marmar, Horowitz, Weiss, Wilner, & Kaltreider, 1988; Vachon, Lyall, Rogers, Freeman-Letofsky, & Freeman, 1980; Walls & Myers, 1985). Despite the small number of systematic studies, we believe they are worthy of review. Some are frequently cited, and familiarity with them provides an impression of the state of the field. They are also relevant to our research project. The studies compare particular forms of group intervention with other forms of group intervention, individual forms of intervention, or nonintervention control conditions.

As noted in Chapter 3, previous group intervention methods have addressed the transitional stage of mourning. Almost all have emphasized support and education as a means of helping persons deal with the tasks of mourning. Most of the participants were experiencing normal as opposed to abnormal reactions to grief. The five studies were also found to share several common features. The subjects in the studies were almost all women, and the loss experienced was the consequence of death, in contrast to separation or divorce, despite the fact that divorce has replaced death as the most likely cause of marital dissolution (Kirkpatrick, 1984). The average age of the widows, according to those studies that provided precise information, was early to mid-50s. Most of the methods were short-term in nature.

The first study is that of Barrett (1978), which was conducted in Los Angeles. The 70 widows in the project were randomly allocated to one of three types of group intervention or to a nonintervention control condition. The group interventions, which were led by a female graduate student in psychology consisted of seven once-weekly 2-hour sessions. They were (1) a self-help group, which focused on practical problems of widowhood, (2) a confidant group, which attempted to establish friendships between pairs of participants by means of intimacy-building exercises and discussion, and (3) a consciousness-raising group, which attempted to increase awareness of women's issues by means of sex role examination and discussion. A large set of 18 outcome measures was assessed before and after therapy and at 14 weeks postgroup. A multivariate analysis, which combined the outcome scores, indicated that all four conditions (treatment and control alike) showed significant change. Some measures evidenced favorable change, for example, an increase in self-esteem. Others showed unfavorable change, for example, an increase in the intensity of grief; and some measures indicated ambiguous change, for example, an increase in negative attitude toward remarriage. However, it was clear that there were almost no advantages for treatment over the control condition. And despite the fact that some of the postgroup impressions of participants were more positive for the consciousness-raising groups than for the self-help groups, the overall findings revealed no differences.

The second study is that of Vachon et al. (1980), which was conducted in Toronto. The 162 widows were randomly assigned to either (1) a widow-to-widow intervention, which initially involved individual contact and eventually group contact in a program that followed the principles of Silverman, or (2) a nonintervention condition. The leaders of the intervention group were themselves widows who were trained in supportive counseling. The primary outcome measure was a 30-item interview instrument known as the Goldberg General Health Questionnaire, which was assessed at 6, 12, and 24 months after the husband's death. At 6 months, items reflecting intrapersonal adaptation (e.g., feeling better) favored the intervention condition. At 12 months, items reflecting interpersonal adaptation (e.g., making new friends) favored the intervention condition, whereas there was now little difference in the intrapersonal area. At 24 months, items reflecting overall psychiatric disturbance favored the intervention condition. More women in the intervention condition had moved from the high-distress to low-distress range. Thus the intervention seemed to accelerate positive change in a progression from intrapersonal to interpersonal adaptation, and, further, to overall protection from psychiatric disturbance.

The third study is that of Walls and Meyers (1985), conducted in Memphis, Tennessee. The 38 widows were allocated to one of three 10-session group interventions: (1) a cognitive restructuring group following Beck's model (1976), which focused on the relationship between thoughts and emotions (e.g., catastrophic thoughts about being alone that lead to fear and loneliness); (2) a behavioral skills group following Lewinsohn's model, which involved assertiveness and social skills training to increase the frequency and enjoyment of pleasant activities; and (3) a self-help group following Silverman's widow-to-widow model, or a nonintervention control condition. In each category there was only one group that was led by a female graduate student in clinical psychology. In addition, a total of 10 dropouts from the four conditions reduced the sample size to 28. A large set of outcome measures including some that were particularly relevant to an intervention condition, such as the Beck Depression Inventory, and some that were general, such as Life Satisfaction, were assessed before and after the intervention (or control period) and at one year following the intervention. There were almost no significant differences in outcome among the four conditions. There was only a trend toward less depression for all subjects. Both the cognitive restructuring group and the behavioral skills group showed a significant decrease in the report of participating in pleasurable activities, whereas both the self-help group and the control condition showed significant increases. Overall, the investigators concluded that the three group-therapy interventions had little effect on adjustment to widowhood.

The fourth study is that of Marmar et al. (1988), which was conducted in San Francisco. The 61 widows were randomly assigned to either (1) individual dynamic psychotherapy (12 once-weekly sessions with an experienced therapist), or (2) a mutual-help group intervention following Silverman's principles (also 12 once-weekly sessions, but with a lay widow leader). Unfortunately, the dropout rates were high. The individual therapy intervention lost 32% of its patients prior to completion, and the group intervention lost 77%. Nevertheless, the investigators succeeded in getting most of the widows (both completers and dropouts) back for follow-up evaluation. A large set of outcome measures was assessed at pretherapy, posttherapy, 4 months posttherapy, and 12 months posttherapy. The results indicated that both forms of intervention were associated with significant reduction in key symptoms, with little difference between the two forms. The greatest changes concerned symptom reduction, in contrast to adaptation at work or interpersonal functioning, which showed up later at 4 and 12 months posttherapy, rather than immediately following therapy.

The fifth study is that of Lieberman and Videka-Sherman (1986). It differs from the previous four studies in that it involved a large-scale questionnaire survey of participants and nonparticipants of an international self-help organization called THEOS (They Help Each Other Spiritually), which serves widows and widowers. The organization sponsors a number of educational, social, and supportive group activities. The findings are based on 466 widows and 36 widowers who completed and returned a set of questionnaires initially and again one year later. A variety of standard and tailored outcome measures were included. In one main comparison, THEOS participants from the survey were compared to a separate, nonparticipant, normative control group. Using a multivariate analysis that combined outcome measures, THEOS participants evidenced significantly greater favorable change. In a second main comparison involving only the 502 subjects who had been surveyed, the greater the extent of social participation in the program, the better the outcome. Whereas these findings were viewed as supporting the efficacy of the THEOS program, one major methodologic flaw in the study casts a shadow of doubt over the results. The subjects were not randomly allocated to conditions. Quite to the contrary, they were self-selected. Thus those who chose to participate may have been quite differen from those who did not. In fact, it was reported that the THEOS participants were significantly more distressed initially than the nonparticipants. Although some statistical adjustments were made, they can not eliminate the potential for confounding the conclusions because of initial differences.

Although it was not presented as part of a completed study, Yalom and Vinogradov (1988) reported their experience conducting bereavement "support groups" that included behavioral techniques. The method used included structured exercises such as bringing a picture of the deceased spouse, or the more cognitive exercise of anticipating regret near the termination of the group. The authors intended the group to focus on the difficulties of the transitional stage of the normal grief reaction. They deliberately did not choose typical mental-health clinic patients. Rather, they aimed for a general population of bereaved spouses of cancer patients at least 5 months after the death. In general, they reported a positive experience.

IMPLICATIONS OF GROUP
INTERVENTION STUDIES

Consideration of the cumulative results of the five studies leads one to the conclusion that the findings concerning the efficacy of group intervention methods with the bereaved are not impressive. Of the four clinical trial studies, only the Vachon et al. study and the Marmar et al. study provide positive results. The Vachon study may reflect only an acceleration of eventual, naturally occurring changes, and the Marmar study lacks a control condition. In addition, the positive results from the Lieberman survey are suspect because of initial differences among the participants and nonparticipants. Should one therefore conclude that group interventions are ineffective with the bereaved? We think not. At the same time, though, one should not conclude that they are effective. As frustrating as this may be, the proper conclusion appears to be that the hypothesis has not been adequately tested. Serious limitations in methodology have characterized most of the studies.

Investigators of group intervention methods for the bereaved, like other researchers who look for effective treatments in the mental health field, have an interest in discovering significant differences among various techniques. Therefore, it is somewhat ironic that investigators, by their choice of methodology, have often greatly reduced their chances of finding significant differences in clinical trial studies. The point that we are making is somewhat different from the one usually made by reviewers of intervention techniques for the bereaved. As an example, Alexander (1988) made the following observation and conclusion:

The range of identifiable methods of intervention for the bereaved is increasing. It is not enough, however, merely to introduce new methods; what is also required is a determina-

tion to assess the efficacy of different methods of intervention
and to isolate their critical ingredients. (p. 862)

We agree with Alexander and believe that investigators who show
such determination should be commended. However, we also wish to
add that the use of weak methodology in an attempt to assess the
efficacy of different interventions is not good enough. Weak methodology can lead to misleading conclusions, and misleading conclusions
can be worse than no conclusions at all if they remain unchallenged,
which often seems to happen.

The presence of weak methodology in studies is not due to an
absence of information about what constitutes good methodology. A
number of substantive reviews that address methodology in the psychotherapy research field have been published in recent years. These
include works by the American Psychiatric Association Commission
on Psychotherapies (1982), Garfield and Bergin (1986), and Williams
and Spitzer (1984). Compromises in methodology are usually related
to inadequate resources and/or impatience. Conducting a proper clinical trial of group intervention, or any other type of treatment, requires
a considerable investment of time and resources. An entire team of
referrers, assessors, therapists, and researchers is usually required.
Pressures to economize, that is, to cut corners, are often strong. However, the price of such economizing, which is failure to provide an
adequate test, would seem to be greater, not only to the researchers but
to the discipline of group psychotherapy as a whole.

In the five group intervention studies that were reviewed, several
serious weaknesses in methodology are apparent in one or more of the
studies. One of the primary shortcomings is inadequate sample size.
Sample size is directly related to statistical power, which is the ability
of a statistical test to detect a difference when a difference exists. When
each condition of a study includes only one or two intervention groups
and correspondingly only 10–15 subjects, as some of the studies reviewed did, it becomes extremely difficult statistically to detect significant differences. Large differences among the effects of the group
interventions would have to exist for the statistical test to indicate
significance. Sometimes, small to moderate effects are clinically important. If the sample size is small, such effects will go unnoticed.

A second weakness that can lead to similar problems is the absence
of high initial levels of patient disturbance on outcome measures. This
was the case in some of the studies reviewed, given the nonclinical
nature of the populations that were studied. If large improvements are
not possible, then differences in improvement among the various
conditions studied will be difficult to detect. Again, a conclusion of

"no differences" may be misleading. A third weakness is the presence of differences among conditions on variables other than group intervention. Such differences can serve to confound the results. Thus, in the Lieberman and Videka-Sherman study (1986), differences on initial level of patient disturbance were noted. In some of the other studies, even though a random method of allocation to conditions was used, equivalence among conditions was not guaranteed, owing to small sample size. Matching on potentially confounding variables prior to random assignment is recommended when sample sizes are not large. Finally, a fourth weakness is the use of inexperienced therapists (leaders). Some of the studies reviewed used trainees. Group intervention methods are quite demanding and require clinical skill. The use of experienced therapists increases the likelihood that the group intervention methods will be applied skillfully and that intended technical differences among conditions will be present. Additional weaknesses could be highlighted (Piper, 1988), but those mentioned serve to illustrate the point that inadequate methodology, by itself, can prevent the emergence of significant findings in group intervention studies.

Being aware of the problems associated with compromises in methodology just mentioned, we planned a controlled, clinical trial investigation of our method of time-limited, short-term group psychotherapy for patients suffering from person loss. In choosing the design and procedures for the study, we attempted to give ourselves a better chance of detecting significant treatment effects than some of the previous investigators had provided for themselves. In regard to the four methodologic weaknesses described above, we chose (1) a large sample size, (2) a patient population with clinical levels of disturbance, (3) a method of allocation to conditions that involved matching and randomization, and (4) a set of experienced therapists to lead the groups. In addition, we attempted to incorporate a number of other methodologic features that appear to have received a consensus of support in the literature (Piper, 1988). These included use of a therapy manual to enhance standardization of technique, use of a process analysis system to verify the integrity of technique, use of patient personality measures to investigate patient selection characteristics, and use of a large battery of outcome measures to provide a comprehensive assessment of possible effects. The measures of patient personality and therapy process also allowed us to investigate particular interaction effects and the relationship of process to outcome. The research project will be presented in the next chapter.

CHAPTER **8**

Clinical Trial Project: Outcome Findings

This chapter presents our controlled clinical trial investigation of dynamically oriented, short-term group therapy for loss patients. Emphasis is placed upon the basic outcome findings. If one focuses on the patients, the study may be viewed as an attempt to discover a treatment technique that will lessen the suffering associated with person loss. The scarcity of such research, in particular methodologically strong research, was noted in the preceding chapter. If one focuses on the intervention method, the study may be viewed as an attempt to test the effects of dynamically oriented, short-term group therapy. There has also been a scarcity of research evaluating this particular form of psychotherapy. Poey (1985) observed that "at the present time there is a paucity of rigorous outcome research available on short-term dynamic group psychotherapy even though many such groups are being run" (p. 332).

Interest in the use of short-term dynamic group therapy has paralleled, and to some degree followed, interest and enthusiasm for short-term dynamic individual therapy. In the last 20 years there has been a considerable amount of activity regarding the development and application of short-term therapies, both group and individual. This activity has stemmed from a number of factors, some being more practical and economical in nature and some more conceptual and technical.

With regard to practical and economic factors, there has been concern about the costs of long-term therapies, particularly among third-party payment sources such as governments and insurance companies. In the United States health maintenance organizations and other similar associations have responded by setting limits on the total number of sessions a patient may attend each year. Also of significance is the limited number of practitioners relative to the demand for services. Briefer therapies, particularly group therapies, could allow therapists to treat greater numbers of patients during a given period of time and/or devote more time to other important activities, for example, training, research, and administration, which frequently are neglected. Toseland and Siporin's (1986) general review of the group therapy literature revealed that approximately two thirds of the studies published between 1965 and 1985 concerned the use of group therapies of less than 20 sessions.

With regard to conceptual and technical factors, short-term psychotherapy has allowed dynamically oriented therapists to retain concepts with which they are familiar. It has also stimulated them to become more technically innovative. Short-term psychotherapy has presented a challenge to several long-standing beliefs that have characterized traditional therapies, for example, that the therapist's overt role should largely be passive, that transference interpretations should not be made until the patient and therapist have established a strong working alliance, and that a gradual prolonged period of working through is a requirement of any effective therapy. Although some of these beliefs were questioned by early figures in the field of psychoanalysis (Alexander & French, 1946; Ferenczi & Rank, 1925), a widespread challenge to the theory of analytic technique did not occur until the mid-1970s. Since then a large number of articles and books have been devoted to the topic of short-term psychotherapy. Practitioners have appeared to be receptive to an approach that may prevent some of the dangers inherent in long-term therapies, such as the patient's defensive dependence and undue resistance.

Most reviews of the group therapy literature that have focused on questions of effectiveness have been positive about the potential usefulness of short-term group therapies (Imber, Lewis, & Loiselle, 1979; Kaul & Bednar, 1986; Klein, 1985; MacKenzie, 1990; Poey, 1985). In the case of short-term, dynamic therapy groups, Goldberg, Schuyler, Bransfield, and Savino (1983) provided a very favorable clinical report concerning their work with such groups in Hartford. A similar impression was conveyed by Budman, Randall, and Demby (1981) concerning an uncontrolled outcome study that they conducted in Boston. In recent years positive endorsements such as these have frequently been made at professional conferences in Canada and the United States.

In contrast, a review of the research literature reveals very little in the way of systematic controlled or comparative outcome studies of short-term, dynamic group psychotherapy. Budman, Demby, Feldstein, and Gold (1984) conducted a controlled study that involved two therapy groups (16 patients) and a comparable number of wait-list control patients. Treated patients reported significantly greater improvement regarding their target objectives than did control patients when ratings were taken soon after therapy had ended. However, this difference was no longer statistically significant after a 6-month follow-up period. Two other studies compared short-term, dynamic group therapy to other forms of therapy (LaPointe & Rimm, 1980; Piper, Debbane, Bienvenu, & Garant 1984). Although significant pre–post improvement for short-term, dynamic group therapy was found on a number of outcome scores, it was not found to be superior to the other forms of therapy. In the latter study its results were actually the poorest of the four forms of therapy studied. In summary, one must conclude that the enthusiasm that some clinicians have shown for short-term dynamic group therapy does not rest on a secure foundation of systematic studies.

The primary purpose of our controlled clinical trial was to study the effectiveness of our particular application of short-term, dynamic group therapy for loss patients. We believe that there continues to be a need for such studies. However, we also agree with Kaul and Bednar (1986) in their overview of empirical studies in the group field. They caution researchers about conducting studies that only deal with the effectiveness question. To determine that a particular form of therapy works is an important first step. To discover how an effective therapy works, that is, to elucidate its mechanisms, is a more important long-term objective. Two approaches to finding answers to the "how" question involve the study of patient characteristics (patient suitability criteria) and the study of therapy process in outcome investigations. By focusing on patient characteristics one assumes that some patients are better suited for particular forms of therapy than other patients. By studying therapy process one postulates that certain events have to transpire in therapy to bring about optimal outcome. The two topics are related, insofar as certain patient characteristics facilitate certain kinds of therapy process.

In our clinical trial a patient characteristic of central interest was the personality variable known as psychological mindedness. We used a newly developed measure of the variable (McCallum & Piper, 1990). Operationally we defined psychological mindedness as the ability to identify dynamic components and relate them to a person's difficulties. A complete presentation of the measure and its empirical relationships within the clinical trial is reserved for Chapter 9, since the primary focus of the present chapter is on the effects of therapy per se. A process variable of major interest was the concept known as psychodynamic work. It was also assessed by a newly developed measure known as the Psychodynamic Work and Object Rating System (Piper & McCallum, 1989; Piper & McCallum, in press). Psychodynamic work was operationally defined as the attempt to understand the problems of one or more members of the group, or the group as a whole, in terms of conflict among dynamic components. A presentation of this measure and its empirical correlates is also deferred to Chapter 9. In the present chapter its use as a means of verifying the nature of technique is presented. For example, when the concept of psychodynamic work is applied to the therapist's statements, it provides a measure of interpretation.

The two main hypotheses associated with the therapy technique were:

1. Treated patients will evidence greater benefits than wait-list control patients.
2. Benefits will be maintained 6 months after the termination of therapy.

OVERALL DESIGN AND PROCEDURE

Following a routine procedure, patients who presented to the Walk-in Clinic were initially assessed by 1 of 15 staff therapists and then by 1 of 6 supervisory psychiatrists. When a patient was judged as being suitable for the Loss Group Program, the staff therapist explained the clinical and research procedures to the patient and obtained his or her informed consent. The staff therapist then notified the research coordinator, who contacted the patient to arrange for a 3-hour research assessment. The patient was first assessed for psychological mindedness (PM). The assessment provided a 9-point rating, which allowed patients to be classified as high (5 and higher) or low (4.5 and lower) on PM. Next, a second independent assessor, who was blind to the PM classification, conducted the interview measures of outcome variables. Then the patient completed the questionnaire measures of the outcome battery. After the initial research assessments were finished, the research coordinator matched patients in pairs. The matching criteria were level of PM (two highs or two lows), gender, and age. The coordinator then randomly assigned one member of the pair to the immediate treatment condition and the other member to the wait-list (delayed treatment) control condition. As the pairs accumulated and the two groups (immediate, delayed) began to form, the coordinator additionally attempted to keep the number of high-PM and low-PM patients equivalent in each group. Each therapist was always assigned a matched pair of groups. The therapist first treated the immediate group and then the delayed group. The project included 8 matched pairs of groups, that is, 16 therapy groups in total. The design is presented in Table 8.1.

PATIENTS

A total of 154 patients completed their initial assessments and were assigned to either the immediate or delayed treatment condition. A number of patients dropped out at various times during the study. Some patients (decliners) changed their mind before starting therapy. Others (therapy dropouts) began therapy but left prematurely, that is, before their group ended. Ambivalence about beginning and continuing is common in therapy groups, and the short-term loss groups were no exception. If a patient dropped out early during a particular stage of the study, for example, after one therapy session, the research coordinator attempted to replace the patient with another matched patient. In group therapy, research dropouts affect not only their own future but also that of other patients, owing to the threat that their departure poses to the viability of the group. Both clinical and research requirements need to be coordinated. In the current project, new additions to a therapy group were made until the third therapy session.

During the first 3-month period of the design, the immediate treatment condition suffered 32 dropouts (13 decliners, 19 therapy

TABLE 8.1. Design for Controlled Clinical Trial

Patients	Three-month period	6 (or 3)-month period	6-month period
High and low psychologically minded patients	Short-term dynamic group therapy (immediate)	Follow-up period	
	or	or	
High and low psychologically minded patients	Wait-list control period	Short-term dynamic group therapy (delayed)	Follow-up period

dropouts) out of 68 patients. That represented 47.0% of the patients assigned to the immediate condition. The delay period condition also suffered 32 dropouts (32 decliners), but out of a pool of 71 patients. That represented 45.1% of the patients initially assigned to the delayed treatment condition. Thus the dropout percentages for the immediate (47.0%) and delayed (45.1%) treatment conditions during the first 3-month period were nearly identical. An additional 15 patients were added late in the delay period or just before the delayed treatment groups started to insure sufficient numbers for the therapy groups.

A total of 109 patients actually started in one of the therapy groups (55 immediate treatment, 54 delayed treatment). Of those, 33 (19 immediate treatment, 14 delayed treatment) were therapy dropouts. Thus the overall therapy dropout percentage was 30.3% (34.5% immediate treatment, 25.9% delayed treatment). The therapy dropout percentages for immediate and delayed treatment did not differ significantly.

For the outcome analyses that compared the patients in the immediate treatment condition with the patients in the delay period, 94 patients (42 immediate patients, 52 delay patients) provided pre–post outcome data. The descriptive information about the patients in the study that follows is based on this sample of 94 patients, because they were the primary sample for the outcome analyses. The sample consisted of 68 women and 26 men. Their average age was 36.0 years (SD = 9.3, range = 18–57). Over two thirds (68%) of the patients did not live with a partner, being either widowed (14%), separated (13%), divorced (21%), or single (20%). Most (85%) had at least a high school education, whereas over a quarter (29%) had attended or were attending a technical college and almost one third (32%) had attended or were attending university. Most (80%) of the patients were either employed, responsible for a household, or involved in full- or part-time studies.

All patients had been assessed as experiencing a pathologic grief reaction following the loss of a person through death (29%), separation/divorce (12%), or both types of losses (59%). Because treatment was not crisis intervention, the patients were beyond the initial period of shock and mourning. A list of significant losses was compiled for each patient. For all losses the average length of time since the loss was 6.8 years (SD = 5.3, range = 0.2–19.2). The average age of the patient at the time of the loss was 29.4 years (SD = 9.0, range = 10–53).

Depressive symptomatology, social isolation, loneliness, and low self-esteem were common presenting features. In terms of the

DSM-III (American Psychiatric Association, 1980) the most common Axis I diagnoses were major depression (45%), adjustment disorder (16%), dysthymia (10%), and anxiety disorder (9%). Fourteen percent also received an Axis II diagnosis, usually dependent disorder (11%). Patients manifesting problems of suicidal intent, psychosis, addiction, sexual deviation, sociopathic behavior, or who were currently involved in another form of psychotherapy were excluded from the study. Sixty-nine percent of the patients had had previous contact with a mental health professional, but only 11% had previously received psychotherapy. Interviews with the patients after the immediate treatment or delay period revealed that 46% of the patients had taken psychotropic medication during the initial 3-month period of the present study. In almost all cases (95%) this involved antidepressant medication. The interviews also revealed that 12% had become involved in another type of psychotherapy during the same initial 3-month period.

THERAPISTS

The therapists in the study were a 34-year-old male psychologist; a 32-year-old female psychologist; and a 31-year-old female social worker. They possessed substantial experience with psychodynamic psychotherapy (8, 4, and 4 years respectively). Their experience included conducting initial assessment interviews, long-term and short-term forms of individual and group therapy, and family and couple therapies. The theoretical orientation of all therapies was psychodynamic, although specific techniques were modified for particular populations; for example, marital therapies utilized a systemic–dynamic approach. Their average annual percentage of direct patient contact in the clinic was 55%.

Six months prior to the study, the therapists were further prepared for conducting the groups. They began attending an ongoing weekly training seminar in which conceptual and technical aspects of STG were discussed, and a technical manual and audiotapes of sessions from the pilot and subsequent groups were used. In addition, all group sessions were observed from behind a one-way mirror by the principal investigator to ensure technical adherence and to offer ongoing supervision. The two female therapists conducted six groups each, and the male therapist conducted four. Each therapist conducted an equal number of groups from the immediate and delayed treatment conditions since groups were always assigned in pairs according to the research design.

THERAPY

The conceptual and technical orientation of therapy as described in Chapter 5 was psychoanalytic, that is, based on the notion that recurrent internal conflicts whose components are largely unconscious serve to perpetuate maladaptation. Conflicts concerning the issues of independence versus dependence and intimacy versus primacy in the context of loss were commonly examined. The objective of therapy was to help patients solve their presenting problems by achieving insight into the ways their difficulties were related to unresolved intrapsychic conflicts, hence, initiating a process of working through that would continue beyond the treatment sessions. The technical orientation emphasized an active therapist role in which interpretation and clarification were emphasized over support and direction. Relevant here-and-now events in the group including transference were highlighted and explored. Patients were encouraged to contribute to the therapeutic process of other patients.

A number of procedures serve to enhance the integrity of a particular form of therapy. These include choosing therapists with relevant training and experience, using a technical manual, monitoring the therapy sessions, reviewing the therapy sessions, and providing feedback to therapists. Although these procedures are helpful, they do not guarantee therapy integrity. Verification requires a process analysis of a substantial amount of therapy session material. This is a time-consuming procedure. Raters need to be trained to use a process system reliably before the actual ratings are performed. Demonstration of therapy integrity is essential if others are to understand a study's findings, to be able to compare the technique to those used in previous studies, and to replicate the technique in future studies.

As noted above, the Psychodynamic Work and Object Rating System (PWORS) was used to analyze therapy process in the clinical trial. A statement-by-statement analysis of a substantial amount of material was rated (45 minutes from seven sessions from 12 groups). Details of the system and procedures will be presented in Chapter 9. Relevant to the verification of therapy integrity, the PWORS analysis indicated that the therapist spoke 14% of the time, whereas the average speaking time per patient was 17%. Thus the therapist was nearly as active as the average patient. The analysis also revealed that 84% of the therapist's speaking time was categorized as providing interpretations. Within these interpretations the distribution of conflictual dynamic components addressed by the therapist was as follows: wishes (22%), anxiety (20%), defenses (34%), and other dynamic expressions (i.e., affects, behaviors, and cognitions) (24%). The distribution of objects addressed was: individual patients (47%), subgroups (4%), the group as a whole (39%), and the therapist as a transference figure (10%). The percent of interventions that revealed the therapist personally (i.e., a self-disclosure) was zero. The analysis confirmed that the therapists were active and interpretive, and in addition placed major focus upon both the group as a whole and individuals. A lesser but definite focus was placed upon the therapist as a transference figure. The therapists successfully avoided personal disclosures. Thus the PWORS analysis confirmed that the technique of short-term, dynamic group therapy had been carried out as planned.

OUTCOME VARIABLES

The selection of outcome criteria in psychotherapy studies has always been a difficult and controversial task. Considerable differences in the content of the variables, rating sources, instrument types, and assessment periods exist among outcome studies. This has led to the frequent problem of not being able to compare results from one study to another because the outcome criteria differ so much. In a field where systematic, well-designed studies are few and where studies often take considerable time to complete, it is crucial that investigators be able to capitalize on each other's work in building a cumulative store of knowledge. In response to this and other related concerns, a special section of the National Institute of Mental Health (NIMH; Washington, D.C.) reviewed outcome criteria for adult, outpatient psychotherapy and recommended a battery of measures for use in subsequent studies (Waskow & Parloff, 1975). Their recommendations concerning choice of outcome criteria are consistent with other well-known and highly regarded monographs on this topic, for example, Lambert, Shapiro, and Bergin (1986). The current consensus is that researchers should include a wide range of outcome criteria in their studies. This inclusive approach is based on the notion that change as a result of psychotherapy is multidimensional. Therefore, investigators should monitor outcome from a variety of perspectives. In this way an outcome battery would include variables that are believed to be most sensitive to the treatment techniques being studied and additional variables for which unanticipated effects may be discovered. This approach is based on the strategy that in a relatively young and developing field, one can afford to be somewhat overinclusive in choosing dependent variables, in this case outcome criteria.

The choice of measures for the outcome battery was influenced by the monographs and articles cited above and our own experience in studying and treating psychiatric outpatients. A number of different areas were represented. These included interpersonal functioning, psychiatric symptomatology, self-esteem, life satisfaction, and personalized target objectives. The sources of evaluation included the patient, the therapist, and an independent assessor. Eighteen variables from nine different measures were selected for repeated assessment. They are listed in Table 8.2.

Ten of the variables focused on interpersonal functioning. Of these, six variables were derived from a modified form of the Social Adjustment Scale interview of Weissman, Paykel, Siegal, and Klerman (1971). The interview focused on interpersonal relationships in six areas: work, social (friends), family of origin, sexual, parental, and partner. Two variables were subscales from Hirschfeld, Klerman, Gough, Barrett, Korchin, and Chodoff's (1977) Interpersonal Dependency Inventory. The two variables, which are measured by 32 questionnaire items, are emotional reliance and autonomy. Two other variables came from the Interpersonal Behavior Scale, a 30-item question-

TABLE 8.2. Outcome Measures and Variables

Measure	Variable
Social Adjustment Scale Interview (Modified)	Work area Social area Family of Origin area Sexual area Parental area Partner area
Interpersonal Dependency Inventory	Emotional Reliance Autonomy
Interpersonal Behavior Scale	Present Functioning Present–Ideal Discrepancy
Symptom Checklist 90	Global Severity Index
Beck Depression Inventory	Depression
Impact of Events Scale	Intrusion Avoidance
Rosenberg Self-esteem Scale	Self-esteem
Life-satisfaction Scale	Life-satisfaction
Target Objectives	Severity rated by patient Severity rated by independent assessor

naire that we had previously developed in Montreal (Piper, Debbane, & Garant, 1977). The variables are defined as present level of interpersonal functioning and the discrepancy between present and ideal levels of interpersonal functioning.

Four of the variables focused on psychiatric symptomatology. One variable was the global severity index of the 90-item Symptom Checklist (SCL-90; Derogatis, 1977), which is a rating scale that focuses on nine primary symptom dimensions (Somatization, Obsessive-Compulsiveness, Interpersonal Sensitivity, Depression, Anxiety, Hostility, Phobic Anxiety, Paranoid Ideation, Psychoticism). A principal-components analysis of the nine dimensions yielded one large factor, which was highly correlated ($r(80) = 0.96$) with the Global Severity Index. Thus the global severity index was used to represent the general factor. Another variable was depression as measured by the Beck Depression Inventory (Beck & Steer, 1987). The other two variables came from a measure particularly relevant for the loss patient population, the Impact of Events Scale (Horowitz, Wilner, & Alvarez, 1979). The two variables are the intrusion of unwelcome ideas and the avoidance of themes associated with a traumatic event, such as loss.

The remaining four variables covered several areas. Self-esteem was measured by the 10-item Rosenberg Self-esteem Scale (Rosenberg, 1979). General life satisfaction was measured by a 1-item Life Satisfaction Scale. Finally, the patient and the independent assessor independently rated the severity of disturbance of several target objectives. Prior to therapy the patient, with the help of the independent assessor, formulated a written set of specific nonoverlapping goals, usually between three and five. The severity levels were averaged across the set of objectives for each of the two raters. In addition to covering multiple content areas from several perspectives, the outcome variable battery measured both internal states and overt behavior, both symptomatic complaints and positive interpersonal behavior, and both general areas of functioning and personalized target objectives, which further reflected our intention to be comprehensive. The interview and questionnaire portions of the battery took approximately 60 and 90 minutes, respectively.

BALANCE BETWEEN CONDITIONS ON
POTENTIAL CONFOUNDING VARIABLES

Before making the primary outcome comparisons between the immediate treatment and control conditions, and between the high PM and low PM conditions, we compared the conditions on a number of additional variables to see if they were well balanced. Balance (or equivalence) between conditions is an important issue in psychotherapy research, given the many variables that are capable of influencing outcome. The procedure of matching and randomly allocating patients to conditions is a good method of attempting to achieve balance, but it is not foolproof. If imbalances exist, understanding the meaning of significant differences between conditions can be difficult. In such a situation, differences in outcome might be attributed to the influence of the condition variable (e.g., therapy) and/or the additional imbalanced variable.

Balance between conditions was investigated for six different types of variables. For each type the general class, the variables, and the categories within variables are listed below.

1. *Demographic*: The variables included age, sex (male, female), marital status (single, married, separated/divorced/ widowed), educational status (high school or less, technical or some university, university), and employment status (full-time, part-time, unemployed/retired).
2. *Diagnostic*: The DSM-III Axis I categories included affective disorder, adjustment disorder, other disorder, and no disorder. For Axis II the categories were simply presence or absence of a personality disorder.
3. *Loss*: The variables included the nature of loss (death, separation, both death and separation), the number of losses (one, two, three, or more), the length of time since the loss, and the age at the time of the loss.
4. *Initial Level of Disturbance*: The variables included the initial (pretherapy or predelay) scores for the 18 outcome variables listed in Table 8.2.
5. *Medication*: This variable was defined as the presence or absence of psychotropic medication during the immediate therapy or delay period.
6. *Psychotherapy*: This variable was defined as participation in another type of psychotherapy during the immediate therapy or delay period.

Several types of statistics (chi-square, t test, analysis of variance) were used to test for significant differences between conditions on these variables. The analyses revealed no significant differences between immediate treatment and control conditions or between high-PM and low-PM conditions for the entire set of variables. Thus the design was extremely well balanced on additional variables. The method of patient allocation and the number of patients likely contributed to the high degree of balance achieved.

INDEPENDENT SAMPLE OUTCOME ANALYSES

Three effects were of primary interest. They were the main effect for treatment (immediate treatment vs. control), the main effect for psychological mindedness (high PM vs. low PM), and the interaction of treatment and psychological mindedness. Accordingly, two-by-two ANOVA-type statistics were used to analyze the outcome data. It is common to psychotherapy outcome measures that prescores (pretherapy or predelay) tend to be significantly correlated with postscores (posttherapy or postdelay). Therefore, statistics were chosen that removed the effect of the prescores on the postscores before an examination of the effects of the independent variables (treatment and PM) on the postscores. A statistic that sensitively performs this task is the analysis of covariance. The dependent variable is the postscore and the covariate, whose effect is removed, is the prescore. Given the large number of outcome variables assessed in the study, a multivariate analysis was conducted initially. Only if a multivariate effect (main or interactive) was found to be significant were univariate effects examined. This strategy provided protection against accepting significant univariate effects as important when in fact they might represent chance findings. Whereas a multivariate analysis of covariance (MANCOVA) would appear to have been the appropriate initial step, limitations to the MANCOVA program precluded its use. The program demands that the same covariate (or set of covariates) be used for each dependent variable. In our study the covariate (prescore) is unique to each outcome variable. Instead of the MANCOVA, a nearly equivalent multivariate statistic was used. This was the multivariate analysis of variance (MANOVA), conducted upon residual gain scores for each dependent variable. Residual gain scores represent postscores with the effect of the prescores removed.

A two-by-two MANOVA was conducted using 16 of the 18 outcome variables. Two of the variables (Parental and Partner of the SAS) were excluded owing to low sample size. The MANOVA yielded a significant main effect for treatment, Pillais $F(16,48) = 2.09$, $p < 0.03$. In contrast, the main effect for psychological mindedness and the interaction effect were not significant. Given that a significant multivariate main effect for treatment was found, univariate main effects for treatment were explored. For each of the 16 outcome variables a two-by-two ANCOVA was performed. These results are presented in Table 8.3.

TABLE 8.3. Results of Two-by-Two Analyses of Covariance for 16 Outcome Variables

Outcome measure	n	Treatment effect F	PM effect F	Interaction effect F
Work area (SAS)	79	2.22	2.12	0.32
Social area (SAS)	89	0.02	1.23	0.89
Family area (SAS)	88	3.40[a]	1.54	0.04
Sexual area (SAS)	88	4.61[*]	1.12	0.59
Emotional Reliance	87	0.02	0.30	0.13
Autonomy	87	1.47	0.01	0.48
Present Interpersonal	88	4.84[*]	0.35	2.39
Present–Ideal Discrepancy	87	2.76	0.00	3.38[a]
Global Severity Index	82	13.07[***]	0.06	4.64[a]
Depression	88	12.92[***]	1.31	1.34
Intrusion	87	4.16[*]	0.79	1.49
Avoidance	87	9.69[**]	3.80[a]	0.08
Self-esteem	85	12.07[***]	2.86[a]	5.17[*]
Life Satisfaction	73	9.43[**]	2.01	2.99[a]
Target severity (patient)	82	7.28[**]	0.18	3.97[*]
Target severity (independent assessor)	87	9.43[**]	1.17	3.54[a]

Note. SAS = Social Adjustment Scale; PM = Psychological Mindedness
[a] $p < .10$.
[*] $p < .05$. [**] $p < .01$. [***] $p < .001$.

Significant treatment effects were found for 10 of the variables, and 1 variable approached significance. Inspection of the prescore and postscore means for the 11 variables, which are presented in Tables 8.4 and 8.5, indicated that in all cases treated patients improved more than control patients. Although some significant or near-significant univariate effects for psychological mindedness and the interaction of the two variables were found, they were not further examined owing to the absence of significant multivariate effects.

TABLE 8.4. Results of Pretherapy versus Posttherapy *t* Tests for 16 Outcome
Variables

Outcome variable	*n*	Pretherapy mean	Posttherapy mean	*t*
Work area (SAS)	35	4.7	3.6	4.88***
Social area (SAS)	40	5.0	4.5	1.48
Family area (SAS)	40	4.2	3.4	4.10***
Sexual area (SAS)	39	6.3	4.8	2.60*
Emotional Reliance	40	45.8	43.2	2.30*
Autonomy	40	26.4	27.3	1.31
Present Interpersonal	40	123.5	127.6	1.47
Present–Ideal Discrepancy	40	30.5	29.4	0.53
Global Severity Index	39	1.28	0.66	7.17***
Depression	40	17.6	8.0	5.83***
Intrusion	40	13.5	9.2	3.52***
Avoidance	40	14.5	8.5	4.26***
Self-esteem	42	3.1	2.1	2.73**
Life Satisfaction	41	3.6	4.6	3.75**
Target severity (patient)	40	3.8	2.6	6.13***
Target severity (independent assessor)	40	3.9	2.5	8.29***

Note. SAS = Social Adjustment Scale.
*$p < .05$. **$p < .01$. ***$p < .001$.

In addition to the means, Tables 8.4 and 8.5 include the statistical
results for the examination of change from pretherapy to posttherapy
for treated patients and from predelay to postdelay for control patients. A correlated *t* test was calculated for each variable for each of
the two samples. For treated patients significant improvements were
found for 10 of the 11 variables; for control patients significant improvements were found for 8 of the 11 variables. The occurrence of
significant pre–post changes for untreated control patients is common

TABLE 8.5. Results of Predelay versus Postdelay *t* Tests for 16 Outcome Variables

Outcome variable	*n*	Predelay mean	Postdelay mean	*t*
Work area (SAS)	44	4.5	4.0	1.65
Social area (SAS)	49	5.2	4.5	2.72**
Family area (SAS)	48	4.4	4.0	2.10*
Sexual area (SAS)	49	6.6	6.5	0.27
Emotional Reliance	47	45.2	43.0	2.25*
Autonomy	47	25.3	25.3	0.06
Present Interpersonal	48	126.4	123.3	1.33
Present–Ideal Discrepancy	47	30.6	33.7	0.97
Global Severity Index	43	1.36	1.01	4.11***
Depression	48	20.1	14.4	5.85***
Intrusion	47	15.6	13.3	2.88**
Avoidance	47	14.4	12.9	2.16*
Self-esteem	46	3.0	3.1	0.47
Life Satisfaction	41	3.1	3.6	2.34*
Target severity (patient)	42	3.8	3.2	2.90**
Target severity (independent assessor)	47	4.1	3.2	5.15***

Note. SAS = Social Adjustment Scale.
*$p < .05$. **$p < .01$. ***$p < .001$.

in psychotherapy research. A number of explanations for this phenomenon, which is sometimes called "spontaneous remission," have been discussed in the literature (Campbell & Stanley, 1963). The occurrence of such changes serves to emphasize the importance of comparing changes made by treated patients with changes made by control patients in a clinical trial study. It is not enough to demonstrate significant pre–post changes for treated patients. What needs to be demonstrated is that changes made by treated patients significantly exceed changes made by control patients. In the present project that is what the significant multivariate and univariate (Table 8.3) main effects for treatment demonstrate.

Own-Control Sample Outcome Analyses

Of the 52 patients assigned to the control condition who had provided predelay–postdelay outcome data, 38 patients subsequently completed their therapy group and provided posttherapy outcome data. For these 38 patients it was possible to compare change during the delay period with change during the therapy period. This type of comparison is called an own-control analysis, because each patient serves as his or her own perfectly matched control. For each of the 16 outcome variables, change during the delay period (expressed as a residual gain score) was compared with change during the therapy period (expressed as a residual gain score) by means of a correlated t test. Significantly greater improvement during therapy than during the delay period was found for three of the variables. These were present level of interpersonal functioning from the Interpersonal Behavior Scale, t (32) = 2.99, p < .01; self-esteem, t (32) = 3.02, p < .01; and life satisfaction, t (26) = 2.13, p < .05. This constituted additional evidence that changes made by treated patients significantly exceeded changes made by control patients.

Magnitude of Effect

The outcome results presented thus far have been expressed in terms of statistical significance, which is defined in terms of probability. In reference to the comparison between treatment and control conditions the question is, "What is the probability that the difference in improvement that was observed could have occurred by chance?" If the probability is less than 5 in 100, which represents the conventional $p < .05$ standard, the difference is regarded as significant. Statistical significance is an important criterion. However, like any single criterion, it does not provide all of the information that is important. For example, it does not provide information about the size of impact that one variable has on another. It is a well-known statistical fact that with large sample sizes, relatively small differences between conditions can be statistically significant. In such a circumstance, evidence of statistical significance may be misunderstood to mean evidence of large impact.

In contrast to statistical significance, the criterion known as *magnitude of effect* directly expresses the size of impact that one variable has on another, in our case treatment on outcome. Also in contrast to statistical significance, magnitude of effect has nothing to do with probability. Whereas several mathematical formulas for calculating magnitude of effect exist in the literature, an appropriate one for the present project was provided by Smith, Glass, and Miller (1980). In general they defined magnitude of effect (also called *effect size*) as the difference in average outcome between treated patients and control patients divided by the standard deviation of the control patients. Using this formula with ingredients from the univariate analyses of covariance that we had conducted (i.e., adjusted postscore means and mean square error roots), we calculated an effect size for each of the 16 outcome variables. The results are presented in Table 8.6.

The effect sizes vary considerably from 0.03 for the social (friends) subscale of the Social Adjustment Scale to 0.84 for the global severity index of the SCL-90. All the effect sizes are positive in sign, indicating greater benefit for treated patients. The average effect size for all 16 variables is 0.51. The average effect size for the 10 variables that had significant treatment effects in the ANCOVA analyses was 0.67. They ranged from 0.48 to 0.84. Such effect sizes are usually regarded as moderate-to-large in the psychotherapy literature. Using the language of Smith, Glass, and Miller, an effect size of 0.67 indicates that the benefits of the average treated patient exceeded those of 75% of the control patients. In their own meta-analytic review of controlled psychotherapy studies, which was based upon 1,766 effect sizes from 485 studies, Smith, Glass, and Miller reported an average effect size of 0.85, which indicated that the benefits of the average treated patient exceeded those of 80% of the control patients. The results of the present project were thus similar.

Clinical Significance

A third criterion that differs from both statistical significance and magnitude of effect is *clinical significance*. Clinical significance refers to the clinical importance of an effect. It is possible for the results of a treatment to be both statistically significant and large in effect size and yet be clinically unimportant. Central to the meaning of clinical significance is the consideration of norms. If a patient moves from a pathologic level to a normal level on a particular variable, a clinically significant change has occurred.

Jacobson and Revenstorf (1988) have described several indices that quantitatively represent movement from a pathologic level to a normal value. One procedure involves calculating a clinical cutoff criterion for each outcome variable. In the present project two of the outcome variables, the SCL-90 and the Beck Depression Inventory, had sufficient normative data to calculate such a cutoff criterion. For the

TABLE 8.6. Therapy versus Control Effect Sizes for 16 Outcome Variables

Outcome variable	Effect size	Percentage of control patients exceeded by the average therapy patient
Work area (SAS)	0.35	64%
Social area (SAS)	0.03	51%
Family area (SAS)	0.41	66%
Sexual area (SAS)	0.48	68%
Emotional Reliance	0.03	51%
Autonomy	0.27	61%
Present Interpersonal	0.49	69%
Present–Ideal Discrepancy	0.37	64%
Global Severity Index	0.84	80%
Depression	0.81	79%
Intrusion	0.46	68%
Avoidance	0.70	76%
Self-esteem	0.79	78%
Life Satisfaction	0.79	78%
Target severity (patient)	0.61	73%
Target severity (independent assessor)	0.71	76%
Mean of all 16 variables	0.51	70%
Mean of 10 significant variables	0.67	75%

SCL-90, Derogatis (1977) reported a mean global severity index of 1.26 for 1,002 psychiatric outpatients and a mean of 0.31 for 974 non-patients. Using Jacobson and Revenstorf's formula, the clinical cutoff criterion for the SCL-90 was 0.64. In our project 45% of the patients in the immediate treatment condition and 28% of the patients in the control condition traversed the criterion, that is, moved from the pathologic to the normal range. Viewed in an alternative way, patients in the immediate condition as a group moved from a mean initial level of 1.28 to a posttherapy level of 0.66. Thus they moved about two thirds of the way from the psychiatric outpatient level to the nonpatient level. In contrast, control patients as a group moved from a similar, mean initial level of 1.36 to a postdelay level of only 1.01, or about a third of the way toward the nonpatient norm.

For the Beck Depression Inventory, Beck and Steer (1987) reported a mean of 17.5 for 99 dysthymic patients and a mean of 4.7 for 143 female college students. Using Jacobson and Revenstorf's formula, the clinical cutoff criterion was 8.2. In our project 55% of the patients in the immediate treatment condition and 28% of the patients in the control condition traversed the criterion. Again, viewed in an alternative way, patients in the immediate condition as a group moved from a mean initial level of 17.6 to a posttherapy level of 8.0, whereas patients in the control condition as a group moved from a mean initial level of 20.1 to a mean postdelay level of 14.4.

For both the SCL-90 and the Beck Depression Inventory it is evident that treated patients as a group did not completely reach the mean levels of nonpatients by the end of their 3-month loss groups. Nevertheless, they came considerably closer than patients in the control condition. A similar conclusion can be made regarding the percentages of patients in each of the two conditions who traversed the cutoff criteria for the two outcome variables.

Follow-up Analyses

Patient cooperation in providing 6-month follow-up data was excellent. Assessments were available for 90% (68 of 76) of the patients who had completed either immediate therapy or delayed therapy. The results are presented in Table 8.7. As indicated, four of the variables (work and social functioning according to the SAS, emotional reliance, intrusion) showed significant additional improvement over the follow-up period and two of the variables (avoidance, target objective severity rated by patient) showed near-significant additional improvement. The overall pattern for the 16 outcome variables indicated additional improvement or maintenance of benefits 6 months after therapy had ended.

Examination of Outcome Effects for Several Additional Variables

The impact of three additional variables on outcome was examined statistically. The first two were therapist and use of medication. Whereas previous analyses had demonstrated that the treatment and

TABLE 8.7. Results of Posttherapy versus Follow-up *t* Tests for 16 Outcome
Variables

Outcome variable	n	Posttherapy mean	Follow-up mean	t
Work area (SAS)	58	3.4	3.0	2.47*
Social area (SAS)	63	4.6	4.1	2.08*
Family area (SAS)	62	3.3	3.2	1.35
Sexual area (SAS)	63	5.6	5.7	-0.27
Emotional Reliance	66	43.6	41.1	3.51***
Autonomy	66	26.4	26.4	-0.13
Present Interpersonal	66	127.2	128.2	-0.43
Present–Ideal Discrepancy	66	28.8	27.2	0.78
Global Severity Index	65	0.7	0.7	0.26
Depression	64	9.6	9.6	-0.03
Intrusion	61	9.6	7.2	3.67***
Avoidance	61	8.0	6.5	1.95a
Self-esteem	65	2.1	1.8	1.61
Life Satisfaction	57	4.6	4.4	0.61
Target severity (patient)	61	2.6	2.3	1.88a
Target severity (independent assessor)	60	2.4	2.4	0.73

Note. SAS = Social Adjustment Scale.
a$p < .10.$ *$p < .05.$ ***$p < .001.$

control conditions were balanced on these two variables, it was still
possible that they might have an independent impact on outcome.
There were three therapists who differed on overt characteristics such
as gender and profession. Other differences such as verbal style and
personality were not formally measured but were assumed to exist.
Use of medication referred to taking psychotropic medication, usually
an antidepressant. Each of these two variables was used as an independent variable (three levels for therapist, two levels for medication)

in a multivariate analysis (MANOVA or Hotelling's T^2) with the 8 immediate treatment groups where the dependent variables were the 16 outcome variables. Both were nonsignificant. Thus therapist and use of medication were not found to have a significant impact on outcome. The third variable examined was group. Kaul and Bednar (1986) have argued that each therapy group has unique ecologic features that may have a significant impact on outcome. For example, the composition of each therapy group is the product of a unique combination of individual patients who evolve their own norms and communication patterns. A MANOVA with group (eight levels) as the independent variable and the 16 outcome variables as the dependent variables was conducted. It was also found to be nonsignificant.

SUMMARY OF THE OUTCOME FINDINGS

The results of the clinical trial were clearly supportive of the effectiveness of time-limited, short-term, dynamic therapy groups for patients experiencing difficulties following the loss of one or more persons. Treated patients improved significantly more on a number of outcome variables than did their matched counterparts who had been assigned to a wait-list control condition. The results were evident from both independent sample and own-control comparisons. Of the set of outcome variables that indicated significant differences, some were particularly relevant to the problems of loss patients. These included depression, low self-esteem, and the intrusion and avoidance of thoughts about the lost person(s). The specific target objectives of patients improved significantly more as well. This was verified by both the patient and an independent assessor. Although most of the outcome variables changed significantly more as a result of treatment, not all did. Interpersonal functioning with work associates (SAS Work Area), friends (SAS Social Area) and close associates (Present–Ideal Discrepancy), as well as general interpersonal dependency (Emotional Reliance, Autonomy) did not. Several of these interpersonal variables did not change significantly over the course of treatment. It is possible that such variables require a longer course of treatment than 3 months, or a different type of therapy. Follow-up assessments conducted 6 months after therapy had ended provided encouraging results. In general, benefits were maintained. For several of the variables, including some of the most relevant (e.g., intrusion, avoidance, and target objectives) additional significant or near-significant improvements were reported. The follow-up results suggested that therapeutic processes continued beyond the termination of the therapy groups.

Outcome was also measured in terms of magnitude of effect. The effect sizes for the statistically significant variables ranged from moderate to large and were comparable in size to those reported in meta-analytic reviews of psychotherapy outcome in the literature. Examination of the clinical significance of the results for two outcome variables that had substantial normative data indicated important changes for the treated patients. Overall, the results provided a strong endorsement for the treatment form used.

We believe that the validity of the results is strengthened by the methodology that was used. The project involved a total of 154 patients, who were assigned to either an immediate or a delayed therapy group. As indicated by their presenting difficulties and their initial scores on the outcome variables, they represented a genuine clinical population. A careful method of matching and random assignment was used, which resulted in well-balanced conditions on a large set of potentially confounding variables. Three experienced therapists provided treatment. A detailed process analysis of session material from 12 of the 16 groups revealed that the technique had been carried out as planned. Repeated measurement of a broad range of outcome variables from different sources provided a comprehensive assessment of outcome effects. As suggested previously, we believe that our choice of methodology allowed us a better opportunity to detect benefits associated with short-term group psychotherapy than other investigators of group interventions for the bereaved have allowed themselves. The present study allowed little room for doubt that evidence of substantial benefits was there to be detected.

CHAPTER **9**

Psychological Mindedness and Psychodynamic Work

This chapter focuses on two concepts that are relevant to the process and outcome of all forms of psychoanalytically oriented therapies, including short-term group psychotherapy for loss patients. The first concept is the patient personality characteristic known as *psychological mindedness*; the second is the patient performance characteristic known as *psychodynamic work*. Despite the familiarity of these concepts and the importance attributed to them in clinical settings, their measurement has proven difficult. Furthermore, the number of clinical studies in which they have been investigated is relatively small. Over a number of years we have developed specific measures for the two concepts. The clinical trial outcome study described in the last chapter provided an opportunity to use the measures to test several clinical hypotheses. These involved the relationships among four variables: psychological mindedness, psychodynamic work, remaining, and therapy outcome. For each concept we will offer a definition, followed by a method of measurement and an elaboration of its psychometric properties. Then each concept's relationships with other key variables in the study will be addressed.

PSYCHOLOGICAL MINDEDNESS (PM)

In 1973 Appelbaum wrote: "Different people mean different things by 'psychological mindedness.' Such words as insightfulness, reflectiveness, introspectiveness, capacities for self-observation, self-appraisal and self-awareness are often used synonymously" (p. 35). This type of interchangeability of meaning, which is fairly common in the mental health field, inevitably leads to confusion and poor understanding of psychological concepts. A second problem that has characterized definitions of psychological mindedness, as well as many other concepts in the mental health field, is overloading. This occurs when a concept is defined in terms of a number of components, some of which appear to represent independent concepts. Appelbaum's own definition of psychological mindedness, which is frequently cited, did not entirely escape this problem. To him psychological mindedness referred to "a person's ability to see relationships among thoughts, feelings, and actions, with the goal of learning the meanings and causes of his experiences and behavior" (p. 36). Appelbaum distinguished four independent parts of his definition. In a similar way, recent investigators have appeared to incorporate other psychological components into their definitions and measures of psychological mindedness, for example, effortful cognitive endeavors (Bagby, Taylor, & Ryan, 1986) and motivation (Conte, Plutchik, Jung, Picard, Karasu, & Lotterman, 1990).

A third problem that has contributed to ambiguity regarding the meaning of psychological mindedness is that of indirect measurement. This has been done in two ways. The first, which has characterized some of our earlier work (Piper, de Carufel, & Szkrumelak, 1985) as well as that of others (Rosenbaum & Horowitz, 1983), was obtaining a rating of psychological mindedness along with a number of other concepts from a general clinical appraisal. The second was deriving a measurement of psychological mindedness by combining scores from other variables (Horowitz, 1989; Kernberg, Burstein, Coyne, Appelbaum, Horowitz, & Voth, 1972).

After reviewing previous definitions and measures of psychological mindedness and considering some of the associated problems, we formulated a number of objectives that helped guide the development of our new measure. The objectives included:

1. *A focused definition.* We chose a limited rather than a multifaceted definition of psychological mindedness. We decided to risk excluding some important aspects in order to achieve conceptual clarity and parsimony. We defined psychological mindedness as the ability to identify dynamic (intrapsychic) components and relate them to a person's difficulties. We believe that this definition captures the essence or central features of several of the previous definitions presented in the literature. A crucial aspect of analytically oriented therapy involves developing insight into the ways presenting complaints may be compromise formations of underlying psychic conflicts involving unpermissible wishes, anxiety (or fear), and defense mechanisms

mobilized to cope with anxiety. The patient needs to be capable of considering that current difficulties may be linked to unconscious conflicts.

2. *A direct measure.* We constructed our measure so that the person's verbal response would directly reveal his or her ability to identify and relate the above-mentioned dynamic components. By focusing on overt, verbal referents, we attempted to minimize the amount of inference required to score psychological mindedness. In addition, we attempted to avoid measuring psychological mindedness in terms of a combination of other concepts. A detailed description of the measure will be described below.

3. *A time-efficient measure.* Instead of using a lengthy interview or questionnaire format, we attempted to construct a measure that would be practical for clinical as well as research endeavors. The instructions and procedures for scoring psychological mindedness are relatively simple. The entire assessment typically requires about 15 minutes.

4. *An engaging measure.* Consistent with the current era's affinity for television and video presentations, we chose a videotape measure. We believed that a videotape measure would be more enjoyable and less intimidating to the subject while at the same time reducing researchers' overreliance on paper-and-pencil tests.

PSYCHOLOGICAL MINDEDNESS ASSESSMENT PROCEDURE (PMAP)

The PMAP is individually administered. The videotape presents a simulated patient–therapist interaction. The interaction is portrayed by actors according to scripts developed to reflect various components of psychodynamically oriented therapeutic process. The interaction begins with an actress-patient describing a recent event in her life to her male therapist.

> I don't . . . [*Silence*]. I don't know where to begin. [*Silence*] I feel so weird lately; kind of at loose ends. [*Pause*] It started last week and just won't go away. [*Long pause*] I didn't know if I should even tell you this. [*Silence*] I went shopping last Wednesday and while I was walking through Eaton's, I saw my husband—my ex-husband, I mean. There he was, not ten feet in front of me at the jewelry counter. At first, I just wanted to rush up to him and say "Hi, long time no see—how about lunch or something." But then I thought, well, he's probably buying a present for his new girlfriend and he'd just feel awkward—or maybe he'd think I was spying on

him—or I don't know what. I started to feel really nervous. I felt like I just had to get out of there. I felt like I was back in high school watching this guy I used to have a terrible crush on. It was like I couldn't move or speak—I just stood there, watching. I watched for a long time, daydreaming . . . Oh, I don't know, maybe of how nice it would be if he were buying a necklace for me. He'd come home and I'd be cooking dinner. He'd come up behind me and put it around my neck. I'd be so surprised and happy and everything would be okay again. [*Smiles*] Sometimes I really wish he'd come back. [*Pause. Looks very thoughtful*] But then, I know I'm really better off without him. [*Looks very sad*] God, he was such a—I get so angry when I think of how it used to be—I sometimes wish I had never met him. Oh, I don't know how I feel, I feel so weird.

The patient's statement includes verbalizations reflecting dynamic components (e.g., conflictual wishes and fears, defensive maneuvers, and parallels between internal and external events, that is, links between cognitions/affects and behavior). The statement constitutes the test stimulus for assessing psychological mindedness. After viewing, the tape is stopped, and the person being assessed is asked for his or her general impressions: "What seems to be troubling this woman?" Part 1 is then replayed (in an attempt to eliminate possible confounding effects owing to memory differences among respondents), and the person is allowed to elaborate on his or her initial answer.

The PMAP differentiates nine levels of PM (Table 9.1). The criteria for each level reflect the ability to identify dynamic (intrapsychic) components and to relate them to a person's difficulty. They also reflect basic assumptions of psychodynamic theory. To obtain a high PM score, a person must provide evidence that he or she is able to use several assumptions held by psychodynamic therapists concerning human behavior. The rationale for the hierarchy is that, in general, a higher level is more comprehensive and complex in its focus by virtue of incorporating criteria from the lower levels. The criteria for the higher levels of the scale, based on clinical experience, require more sophisticated and elaborate explanations than those for the lower levels. In addition, the hierarchy reflects a temporal sequence that is consistent with psychodynamic theory (e.g., anxiety develops before defensive maneuvers are deployed).

The criteria for Levels I through III are based on the assumption of *psychic determinism*, whereby all human functioning is assumed to result, at least in part, from an internal or psychic process. For example, the statement "Her loneliness is making her feel depressed" meets Level III criteria by clearly attributing the depression to the internal state of loneliness. Level IV criteria require an understanding of the

TABLE 9.1. The Nine Levels of Psychological Mindedness

Level I	The subject identifies a specific internal experience of the patient.
Level II	The subject recognizes the driving force of an internal experience of the patient.
Level III	The subject identifies a result of a drive such that a causal link is made between an internal event and its resultant expression.
Level IV	The subject recognizes that the motivating force in the patient is largely out of her awareness or is unconscious.
Level V	The subject identifies conflictual components of the patient's experience.
Level VI	The subject identifies a causal link where the conflict is presented as generating an expression.
Level VII	The subject identifies a causal link where tension (fear, anxiety) is presented as motivating an expression.
Level VIII	The subject recognizes that the patient is engaging in a defensive maneuver.
Level IX	The subject recognizes that despite the defensive maneuver, the patient remains disturbed in some way by the conflict.

unconscious. The criteria for Level V, the midpoint of the scale, correspond to the recognition of ambivalence or conflict, or both. A basic assumption underlying the psychodynamic understanding of motivation is that internal impulses (id) come into conflict with the frustrating or nongratifying aspects of external reality or their internalized representatives (superego) while the more rational part of the personality (ego) acts as mediator. An example of a response meriting a Level V rating is: "Well, she wants to be with her husband again, but at the same time she's still very angry with him."

The criteria for Levels VI and VII reflect the assumption that a conflict generates tension and attempts at resolution. The conflicted impulses are permitted expression through compromise formation after being filtered through self-protecting defense mechanisms. This is reflected in the criteria for Level VIII. These attempts are, however, only partially successful. This latter assumption is reflected in the criteria for Level IX. An example of a Level IX rating is: "That's sour grapes to say she's 'really better off without him.' I think she really feels that she'd be a lot happier with him."

To provide case illustrations of how the scoring criteria are used, we will consider the verbatim responses of the two patients who were

described in Chapter 4, Ellen and Margaret. Ellen's response to the
open-ended question, "What seems to be troubling this woman?" was
as follows:

> Well, she was married and now she's divorced. She's just having
> a hard time coping with it. Sounds like he's got another woman.
> Seeing him brings back the past. She wished it was the good times
> again and that makes her sad.

To determine which score her response merits, consider that the criteria for Levels I through III are based on the assumption of "psychic
determinism." Ellen's statement, "She wished it was the good times
again and that makes her sad" attributes the patient's sadness to the
internal motivator of the wish for something from her past, thereby
reflecting the assumption of "psychic determinism." The rest of her
response is not considered to reflect psychodynamic assumptions
beyond Level III. Thus her final psychological mindedness score is 3,
which is clearly in the low range of the scale.

In contrast, consider Margaret's response to the open-ended
question:

> Seeing him again brought back wishful thinking. She realizes it's
> wishful thinking, but it doesn't help. So she's thinking about the
> difficult times, but she still would like it to be the way she wished
> it would be. Not a good feeling to realize that you want somebody
> that you can't have and to know at the same time that if you did
> have him you wouldn't want it. Kind of leaves a person feeling
> confused and scared. She says weird; I think she feels foolish and
> scared about wanting him back so she becomes all reasonable and
> tries to talk herself into not wanting him back but underneath it
> all the feelings are still there. Like when she says husband and then
> corrects herself to exhusband, I had to think she still feels a very
> strong attachment to him.

Like Ellen, Margaret meets the criteria for Levels I–III. Beyond that she
meets the criteria for a number of other levels. The criteria for Level V
correspond to the recognition of ambivalence and/or conflict.
Margaret's statement, "Not a good feeling to realize that you want
somebody that you can't have and to know at the same time that if you
did you wouldn't want it" reflects this assumption, thus meeting the
criteria for Level V. Continuing up the scale, the criteria for Levels VI
and VII, which reflect the assumption that a conflict generates tension
and attempts at resolution, are also met. In addition, Margaret indicates, "Kind of leaves a person feeling confused and scared. She says

weird; I think she feels foolish and scared about wanting him back, so she becomes all reasonable and tries to talk herself into not wanting him back, but underneath it all the feelings are still there." Margaret's response reflects the assumption that the patient's conflicted impulses are permitted expression only after being filtered through a defense mechanism, in this case rationalization. Finally, Margaret recognizes that despite the patient's defensive response, she remains disturbed. Thus criteria for Levels VIII and IX are met. Overall, Margaret receives a score of 9, which is clearly in the high range of the scale.

In summary, the PMAP was developed to be a more objective, direct measure of psychological mindedness. The conceptual definition is more precisely psychoanalytic than some of the earlier definitions. This emphasis was based on the goal of differentiating psychological mindedness from other related concepts (e.g., motivation). It was also based on the hope that by developing a pretherapy measure of PM that assessed the abilities required of work within a psychoanalytically oriented therapy, its predictive ability would be enhanced. The standard stimulus of the videotape allowed for the utilization of scoring criteria that reflected clearly defined behavioral referents. The advantage of a standard stimulus over appraisals based on clinical interviews is the reduced possibility of other variables influencing the PM rating (e.g, likability). In addition, it is a skillful interviewer indeed who can assure a valid rating of PM by devoting sufficient attention to each variable he or she is assessing. Similarly, he or she must create a consistent ambiance so that each patient feels equally at ease discussing his or her problems in a standard amount of time. Other advantages of the videotape method are that it seems to be an enjoyable and nonintimidating procedure, and one that is time-efficient for the person being assessed as well as the assessor.

PSYCHOMETRIC PROPERTIES OF THE PMAP: NONCLINICAL STUDY

The psychometric properties of the PMAP were investigated initially with a nonclinical population in a study conducted in Montreal, Quebec. The subjects, procedure, results, and conclusions of the study are presented next.

Subjects

Adult subjects were recruited to participate in a study on "the perception of psychotherapy," for which they were not paid. The first

30 volunteers (19 women and 11 men) who responded to the recruit-ment notices were accepted. Their mean age was 36.3 years (range = 19–67). Twelve participants were married, 5 were divorced, and 13 were single. Eight of the subjects were either enrolled in or had com-pleted graduate studies (not psychology), whereas the remainder had completed at least 1 year of undergraduate studies. The mean PM score was 6.2, with a standard deviation of 2.5.

Procedure

Using the PMAP, each subject was first assessed for PM. To determine interrater reliability, all responses to the PMAP were au-diotaped. The raters were two female graduate students of clinical psychology who were familiar with analytic concepts. To investigate the construct validity of the PMAP, each subject was asked to provide demographic information and was administered a battery of person-ality measures. To determine test–retest reliability, one half of the subjects were randomly chosen to be reassessed 1 month later on the PM measure.

Two other measures of PM were administered: The Psycholog-ical Mindedness (PY) scale of the California Psychological Inven-tory (CPI; Gough, 1957), and the Insight Test (Tolor & Reznikoff, 1960). The depression and anxiety scales of the SCL-90 (Derogatis, 1977) assessed psychiatric symptomatology. An assessment of ver-bal intelligence was provided by the brief intelligence test called the Quick Test (Ammons & Ammons, 1962). Other measures of person-ality included the Cognitive Structure, Achievement, and Social Desirability scales of the Personality Research Form (PRF; Jackson, 1974)

Interrater Reliability Results

The two raters independently rated the (audiotaped) responses of one half of the subjects to the PMAP. For the two sets of ratings the Pearson product–moment correlation coefficient was $r(13) = .81$, $p < .001$, and the intraclass correlation coefficient was .69, $p < .01$.

Test-Retest Reliability Results

Pearson product–moment correlation coefficients conducted on the data of subjects who were reassessed 1 month later revealed that the test–retest reliability of the measure was $r(13) = .76$, $p < .001$.

Convergent Validity Results

To explore the PMAP's convergent validity, subjects' PM scores were correlated with their scores on the other measures of psychological mindedness. The results of Pearson product–moment correlations indicated that the PMAP was significantly related to both the PY subscale of the CPI, $r(28) = .42$, $p < .05$, and the overall insight score of the Insight Test, $r(28) = .50$, $p < .01$.

Additional Construct Validity Results

To explore additional aspects of the PMAP's construct validity, the relationships between the subjects' demographic characteristics and their PM score were investigated. The results of a Pearson product–moment correlation revealed that PM was not significantly related to age. The results of chi-square analyses indicated that PM was not significantly associated with gender, marital status, employment status, or level of education. Its construct validity was further supported by the finding that it was not significantly related to any of the three scales of the PRF (Cognitive Structure, Achievement, and Social Desirability), the intelligence quotient of the Quick Test, or the anxiety and depression subscales of the SCL-90.

Conclusions

The results from the initial study were promising. The reliability of the PMAP was supported, and the evidence concerning the construct validity of PM was theoretically consistent. The results supported our decision to use the PMAP in our clinical trial outcome study of loss groups.

PSYCHOMETRIC PROPERTIES OF THE PMAP: CLINICAL STUDY

Additional information about the psychometric properties of the PMAP were available from the clinical trial outcome study of loss groups. The information presented next was based upon the first eight groups in the study.

Interrater Reliability

Tape recordings of 15 patients' responses to the PMAP were randomly chosen and rated by a second rater. The Pearson product–

moment correlation coefficient for two raters over the 15 patients was $r(13) = .90$, $p < .001$. The intraclass correlation coefficient was .96, $p < .001$. Hence the interrater reliability that had been determined with the nonclinical population was surpassed with the clinical population.

Test–Retest Reliability

Pearson correlation coefficients were calculated for control patients in the delayed treatment condition. The results indicated that the test–retest reliability for PM over the 3-month period was $r(27) = .59$, $p < .001$. Although significant, this coefficient is somewhat lower than that of the nonclinical population. Perhaps the patients, who had been waiting to enter therapy, were less motivated to do the task a second time, or they may have been indirectly expressing feelings about having had to wait for treatment. Other extraneous factors (e.g., memory differences among patients) may have exerted a stronger influence on the stability of the PM score over the extended interval of 3 months.

A separate but related issue concerned the stability of PM. Change over the treatment period and change over the delay period were each investigated with a correlated t test. Neither was significant, which attested to the stability of the PM score over time, even when exposed to treatment.

Convergent Validity

Following sessions 4, 8, and 12, the therapist was asked to provide ratings for a few patient variables, including level of psychological mindedness. The rating scale ranged from (1) *poor* to (7) *excellent*. The relationship between the (mean) therapist rating of PM and the PMAP rating was determined for all patients who had completed therapy. The Pearson correlation coefficient was $r(40) = .30$, $p < .05$. This association offered clinical validation of the manner in which PM had been operationalized. The coefficient also revealed that the two sources of assessment were not redundant.

Discriminant Validity

In addition to PM, the PMAP also assesses the degree to which a person understands psychodynamic interpretations. Following the assessment of PM, an actor-therapist responds to the actress-patient by interpreting first the dynamic components of her conflict and then the transferential aspects (i.e., her attempt to repeat with the therapist a past mode of interaction). Both types of interpretations are presented in three stages. At each subsequent stage the degree of ambiguity and therefore the degree of difficulty is less. The tape is stopped after each interpretation and the person being assessed is asked "Where is he getting that from?" or "What does he mean by that?" The therapist's responses constitute the test stimulus for assessing Interpretation Comprehension, defined as the ability to identify the referents of therapeutic interpretations. It has three subscores: the Number of Dynamics understood; the Speed of Dynamics, which reflects the ease with which the dynamics are understood; and the Speed of Transference, which reflects the ease with which the interpretation of transference phenomena is understood.

Pearson product–moment correlation coefficients were calculated between PM and each of the three Interpretation Comprehension variables. The results indicated that PM was significantly, but not highly, related to Number of Dynamics, $r(77) = .34$, $p < .01$, and Speed of Dynamics, $r(77) = .25$, $p < .05$, and nonsignificantly related to Speed of Transference, $r(77) = .20$. In the case of the Dynamic variables, the low correlations were not due to low reliability. The intraclass correlation coefficients for Number of Dynamics (ICC = .82, $p < .001$) and Speed of Dynamics (ICC = .83, $p < .001$) were both significant. In the case of Speed of Transference, low reliability (ICC = .47) may have contributed to the low correlation.

These results suggested that the ability to generate a psychodynamic understanding of a person's difficulties (PM) was relatively independent of the ability to understand therapist interpretations of conflict between dynamic components. Although there may be similar (cognitive) processes underlying these two abilities, it is probably more difficult to generate one's own understanding (PM). The rather low reliability of the Transference variable renders the weak relationship between PM and that variable difficult to interpret. Conceptually, transference differs significantly from PM. The former concept refers to a repetitive pattern of relationship, whereas the latter refers to conflictual dynamic components. We believe, therefore, that the low correlations between PM and the Interpretations Comprehension variables indicate that the PMAP's assessment of psychological mindedness is not confounded by the method of assessment, supporting its discriminant validity.

Additional Aspects of Construct Validity

A Pearson product–moment correlation and a series of chi-square analyses reaffirmed, with this clinical population, that PM was not significantly related to age, gender, marital status, employment status, or level of education. In addition, the use of medication and aspects associated with the loss did not differ for patients obtaining high versus low PM ratings. A series of t tests revealed that initial scores on the outcome measures were not significantly related to being rated high or low on PM.

Conclusions

The information obtained from the clinical study concerning the psychometric properties of the PMAP reaffirmed and strengthened the results from the initial nonclinical study. The reliability of the PMAP was again supported, and the evidence concerning the construct validity of PM was again theoretically consistent. Strong psychometric properties increase one's confidence in predictive validity findings. Those findings, which concern the relationship of PM to such variables as work, remaining, and outcome, will be considered after the definition and measure of work are presented.

PSYCHODYNAMIC WORK

Our interest in the concept of work stemmed from several sources. First, we have observed that the term *work* is commonly used in clinical settings to describe valued group activities. The activities are perceived to be instrumental to goal attainment. Second, the term work has been used in several important theories and assessment systems in the field of group therapy. According to Bion (1959), "When patients meet for a group therapy session it can always be seen that some mental activity is directed to the solution of the problems for which the individuals seek help" (p. 144). He called that activity the *work group*. Thelen, Stock, Hill, Ben-Zeev, and Heintz (1954) created a rating system to rate Bion's concept of work. Later Hill (1965), a colleague of Thelen, developed a rating system for group therapy that gave primary attention to the concept of work. It was called the Hill Interaction Matrix. Early findings concerning the system's reliability and validity were promising. However, more recent work with the system, including some of our own, encountered reliability problems. Furthermore, the evidence of predictive validity in regard to therapy outcome has been minimal. Part of the difficulty may lie in the general nature of its definition of work, namely, taking the role of patient and actively seeking self-understanding.

A third reason for our interest in the construct of work was the possibility of establishing a more specific definition that was based upon psychoanalytic concepts and theory (Bienvenu, Piper, Debbane, & De Carufel, 1986). In particular we were interested in using the notion of conflict considered through the dynamic point of view (Fenichel, 1945) to formulate an operational definition of work for group psychotherapy. A similar effort to use psychoanalytic theory to define therapist interpretations had proven to be productive (Piper et al., 1987). However, the application to group therapy was more complex because it involved intragroup conflict, in other words, conflict among patients, as well as the intrapsychic conflict of the individual patient.

PSYCHODYNAMIC WORK AND OBJECT RELATIONS SYSTEM (PWORS)

The PWORS is used to rate each statement by a patient or therapist for the presence of work and reference to objects (persons). Work is defined as an attempt to understand the problems of one or more members of the group, or the group as a whole, in terms of conflict among dynamic components. Dynamic components are internal forces in the group that are part of a conflict in the group. These are three familiar concepts of psychoanalytic theory: wishes, anxiety, and defenses. They are assumed to exert an internal force on one or more members, or the group as a whole, and at some level are opposed. In addition to wishes, anxiety, and defenses, which Malan (1976) referred to as the impulse–defense triad, any affect, behavior, or cognition may serve as a dynamic component if it is presented as an internal force that is part of a conflict. If presented as such, it is called a dynamic expression. As an example of a dynamic expression, guilt would be identified as having a subsequent impact, such as motivating a behavior, while as a resultant expression it would be regarded merely as an affective end-product. Thus each statement by a patient or therapist is examined for the presence of one or more dynamic components. If present, the statement is categorized as work.

Objects refer to people internal or external to the group. If internal to the group, the units are a patient, the therapist, a dyad, a subgroup, or the group as a whole. If external to the group, the units are mother, father, parent, sibling, family, a former or absent member of the group, another specific person, a specific group other than the therapy group, or general classes of people (e.g., men, doctors). Each object that is mentioned in a statement is rated. Object linking refers to the identification of a shared interpersonal process between a unit of the group and two other objects. The other objects may be internal or external to the group.

The components and objects of the PWORS are used to differentiate two levels of nonwork and two levels of work. The first nonwork level, Category 1, contains externalizing statements. These focus on topics that do not involve a unit of the group. If an external object is mentioned, its relationship to a unit of the group is not indicated. For example, "Some people are so involved in the church that they ignore their own families." The second nonwork level, Category 2, contains descriptive statements. They provide or request information about a unit of the group. If an external object is mentioned, its relationship to a unit of the group is also indicated. For example, "You seem to be trying to help everyone, even us in the group."

The first work level, Category 3, contains statements that identify a single dynamic component. For example, "You ask everyone how they feel so you don't have to talk about how you feel." The second work level, Category 4, contains statements that identify two or more dynamic components. For example, "I think you're afraid to feel vulnerable in here, and that's why you pretend to have all the answers." Thus, the two work levels differ only in complexity. The higher level usually indicates a greater appreciation of the conflictual nature of dynamic components.

To use the PWORS, each statement by a patient or therapist from taped group therapy sessions is timed using a stopwatch. A statement is defined as a part of a sentence, a complete sentence, or more than one sentence spoken by a member of the group that is not interrupted by a statement by another member or by silences greater than 10 seconds. For each statement the PWORS determines the category of work, the object focus, and whether or not there is object linking. Participation is the ratio of the patient's total statement duration over the total verbal production of the group. It is the individual's portion of speaking. Self-based work is the patient's work behavior (statements scoring Categories 3 or 4) relative to his or her total participation. It is how much an individual works when he or she speaks. The degree of inference required of a rater for the work–nonwork levels is considerably greater than for objects, which are easily identified. However, by having raters make judgments solely about the presence of dynamic components, which then automatically determine the work level, inference is kept to a manageable degree.

RELIABILITY OF THE PWORS

Interrater reliability was investigated in the clinical trial outcome study of loss groups. Four research assistants with an undergraduate degree in psychology or the equivalent were trained to use the PWORS. The training sessions involved approximately 1 day per week over a 4-month period. Subsequently, 7 of the 12 STG sessions (1, 2, 4, 6, 8, 10, 12) from each of the first 12 groups of the study were analyzed with the system. The aim was to obtain a large data base for all patients from each phase of therapy. The raters listened to the first 30 minutes of each session for context and then rated the next 45-minute segment.

Interrater reliability was determined by comparing pairs of independent ratings of 12 randomly chosen sessions which provided 1,572 statements for categorization. The average percentages of perfect category agreement for Categories 1 through 4 were 87, 83, 67, and 66, respectively. The average kappa coefficient, which indicates the proportion of category agreement between two raters after removing the influence of chance-expected agreement, was .69. The majority of disagreements were between the two nonwork or the two work categories. The raters rarely disagreed about the work–nonwork distinction. Thus, the data supported the reliability of the system.

RELATIONSHIP BETWEEN PSYCHOLOGICAL MINDEDNESS AND REMAINING, WORK, AND OUTCOME

Remaining

The overall pattern of patient attrition for the 154 patients who were assigned to either the immediate or delayed treatment condition in the study is summarized in Chapter 8. As indicated, 109 patients actually started in one of the 16 therapy groups, and the dropout percentage was 30.3%. The dropout percentages for immediate and delayed treatment did not differ significantly. High attrition can be a significant problem in group therapy. For the dropout, further therapeutic work in the group is precluded, and feelings of lack of closure and failure are potentially harmful. Attrition can also disrupt the work of the remaining patients and can be discouraging to therapists. Although not all dropouts represent therapeutic failures (Lothstein, 1978), many do. Unfortunately, high dropout rates are commonly reported in the literature (Baekeland & Lundwall, 1975). If clinicians could identify patients at high risk for dropping out before therapy began, they could take preventive action. This might take the form of special preparation procedures or particular therapist techniques that enhance the alliance or reduce anxiety.

For both practical and theoretical reasons we were interested in examining the relationship between psychological mindedness and remaining. PM represented the patient's ability to identify dynamic components and relate them to a person's difficulties. We believed that the general psychoanalytic orientation of treatment and the particular technical emphasis of the therapist on the interpretation of conflict would require the ability represented by PM. Patients rated high on PM might have an easier time in therapy, whereas patients low on PM might have a more difficult time. High-PM patients were defined as those with a score of 5 or higher on the PM scale; low-PM patients had a score of 4.5 or lower.

A total of 33 of the 109 patients who actually started therapy dropped out prematurely. Twenty-one were early dropouts (attended 1–5 sessions) and 12 were late dropouts (attended 6–8 sessions). In comparing the dropout rates for high-PM and low-PM patients, we found that only 14% (9 of 64 patients) of the high-PM patients were dropouts, whereas 53% (24 of 45 patients) of the low-PM patients were dropouts. The result of a chi-square analysis of these frequency counts was highly significant, $\chi^2(1) = 17.58$, $N = 109$, $p < .001$. The proportion of variance accounted for was .16 (Hudson, Thyer, & Stocks, 1985), indicating a substantial association between PM and dropping out of therapy. Thus our hypothesis was supported.

Following our examination of the relationship between PM and remaining, which had been guided by an a priori hypothesis, we conducted a post hoc search for other pretherapy variables that distinguished remainers and dropouts. We examined a large set of variables, 48 in total, that included demographic characteristics, diagnoses, psychotropic medications, characteristics associated with loss, previous treatments, importance of target objectives, pretherapy scores on outcome variables, and patient expectations of therapy. The research literature contains many studies that list variables such as these that have been found to differentiate dropouts from remainers. However, each study's list of variables tends to be rather unique. In addition, there has been little evidence of cross-validation, which involves identifying predictor variables from an initial sample and then examining their predictive ability in a second independent sample. Requirements for the cross-validation procedure include large samples and the assessment of common predictors. That may explain why the procedure has seldom been used in the group therapy field.

Given the relatively large sample size of our study (76 remainers, 33 dropouts), it was possible to randomly divide the sample into two halves and carry out a cross-validation procedure. The specific list of predictor variables investigated and details concerning the cross-validation procedure are presented in a journal article (McCallum & Piper, in press). In addition to PM, only two of the other 48 variables emerged as significant predictors. These were the patient's initial score on the SCL-90 (a measure of psychiatric symptomatology) and the initial severity of disturbance associated with the patient's target objectives (personalized goals for therapy). Dropouts were less psychologically minded and more disturbed in terms of psychiatric symptomatology and the severity of their target objectives than were remainers. A sequence of multivariate analyses (discriminant function) indicated that the combination of the three predictor variables correctly identified 73% of the remainers and dropouts in the first subsample (one half of the patients) and 67% of the remainers and dropouts in the second (cross-validation) subsample (one half of the patients). Thus, although not all remainers and dropouts were correctly identified, a substantial number were.

Our findings are consistent with the conception that patients who lack the ability required of therapy (low-PM patients in our study) *and* who are highly symptomatic and disturbed by their personal problems are at high risk for dropping out. Stated somewhat differently, Budman, Demby, and Randall (1980) concluded that to remain and succeed in a short-term, dynamically oriented therapy group, "a patient needs to be able to 'speak the same language' (as the other members)" (p. 15). In our groups "speaking the same language" can be taken to mean being psychologically minded.

Psychodynamic Work

The relationship between PM and self-based work (as measured by the PWORS) was investigated by a Pearson product–moment correlation for 58 patients who had completed therapy in the first 12 groups. A significant direct relationship was found, $r(51) = .43, p < .001$. When only the higher level of self-based work (Category 4 of the PWORS) was used, the correlation was even higher, $r(51) = .48, p < .001$. In contrast, the correlation between PM and simple participation (work and nonwork) was not significant. Thus, whereas PM was not predictive of talkativeness in the group, it was predictive of the amount of self-based work, that is, the proportion of time a patient works when he or she talks. The patient's ability to identify dynamic components and relate them to a person's difficulties as manifested in the pretherapy PMAP carried over to the patient's tendency to understand the problems of one or more members of the therapy group, or the therapy group as a whole, in terms of conflict among dynamic components. This finding has implications for the selection of patients for psychodynamically oriented group therapy. By choosing patients who are psychologically minded, a group could be primed for the facilitation of psychodynamic work.

Therapy Outcome

The relationship between PM and therapy outcome for all patients in the clinical trial outcome study, that is, patients receiving immediate therapy and patients in the wait-list delay condition, was reported in Chapter 8. The main effect for PM in the multivariate analysis (MANOVA) was not significant. Thus PM was *not* found to be a significant, general prognostic predictor for loss patients. It was possible, however, that PM might be an important predictor variable for treated patients—those who were treated immediately and those who were treated after the wait-list delay period. To test that possibility an additional set of analyses was conducted with all treated patients in the study.

The relationship between PM and therapy outcome for treated patients was investigated with a set of partial and Pearson product–moment correlations. The partial correlation statistic was used with the 18 outcome variables that were measured both before and just after therapy ended. It removed the effect of the before-therapy score prior to determining the correlation between PM and the after-therapy score. The Pearson correlation statistic was used with two global rating measures that were assessed only after therapy ended. They were the ratings for the overall usefulness of therapy according to the patient and the therapist. None of the 20 correlations between PM and therapy outcome were statistically significant.

RELATIONSHIP BETWEEN PSYCHODYNAMIC WORK AND OUTCOME

Like the previous analyses involving PM, the relationship between work and therapy outcome was investigated by a set of partial and Pearson product–moment correlations. The partial correlation statistic, which was used with the 18 outcome variables that were measured both before and after therapy, removed the effect of the before-therapy score prior to determining the correlation between the PWORS, self-based work variable, and the after-therapy score. The Pearson correlation statistic was used with the two rating measures for overall usefulness of therapy that were used after therapy ended. These analyses were based on the 58 patients who had completed therapy in the first 12 groups. There were three significant correlations and three that approached significance. All indicated a positive relationship between work and favorable outcome. They included the family of origin, $r(47)$ = .34, p < .05, and the parental, $r(36)$ = .48, p < .01, subscales of the Social Adjustment Scale interview; the therapist's global rating of overall usefulness, $r(56)$ = .27, p < .09; the independent assessor's rating of target objective severity, $r(47)$ = .25, p < .09; and the patient's global rating of overall usefulness, $r(53)$ = .23, p < .09. Thus there was some evidence, beyond what could be expected by chance, for a direct relationship between self-based work and favorable outcome. The relationship between simple participation and outcome was also investigated. Only one of the 20 correlations was significant (p < .05). Because this is approximately what could be expected by chance, it was concluded that there was no important relationship between participation and therapy outcome.

Although the strongest results were found for self-based work, it is clear that these are in need of replication before they can be accepted as valid. Presently there is only a suggestion of a direct relationship between self-based work and favorable outcome. There are several likely reasons why the correlations were not higher. First, there was a strong, positive treatment effect in the study, and the sample of patients who provided substantial session material for PWORS analyses were completers of treatment. Thus outcome was limited to the good-to-excellent range for most of the sample, which likely served to restrict the possibilities of obtaining high correlations. This, of course, was also true for the correlations between PM and outcome. Second, the PWORS is limited to assessing overt verbal signs of psychodynamic work during the sessions. Psychodynamic work that occurred silently during the sessions or that occurred outside the sessions was not assessed. Third, many other variables, either by themselves or in combination, are capable of influencing treatment outcome. Bloch and Crouch (1985) previously identified three large sets of such variables (conditions for change, therapist technique, and therapeutic factors). Because of this complexity it is unrealistic to expect strong direct relationships between single therapeutic factors such as psychodynamic work and outcome. Fourth, as Stiles (1988) recently noted, patients may require different amounts of therapeutic factors in order to achieve similar goals. The challenge in this case is to identify which patients require which amounts of the factors. That challenge plus the consideration of more complex, interactive models will likely preoccupy investigators for a long time to come.

CONCLUSIONS

This chapter has focused on the relationships among several different kinds of variables. Psychological mindedness is a patient personality characteristic. Accordingly, it was assumed to be a relatively stable characteristic. The analyses that examined change in PM over the treatment period and over the delay period in our clinical trial outcome study confirmed its stability. The variables *psychodynamic work* and *remaining* capture aspects of patient behavior during the course of therapy; they convey information about the process of therapy. The variable *therapy outcome* is a multifaceted one that represents a number of areas of desirable change. In addition, and in contrast to PM, outcome measures were chosen that were believed to be sensitive to the influence of the therapy.

By including different kinds of variables in the study our intention was to learn something about how therapy works and with whom, in addition to whether it is generally helpful. As indicated in Chapter 8, reviewers such as Kaul and Bednar (1986) have cautioned researchers against conducting studies that deal only with the effectiveness question. By choosing patient personality and process variables that were conceptually relevant to the form of therapy being studied, that is, dynamically oriented group psychotherapy, we hoped to enhance our chances of elucidating some of the mechanisms involved in bringing about desirable change. To a certain extent we believe that we have accomplished this objective.

The findings that are most suggestive of underlying mechanisms concern the relationships of psychological mindedness to working and remaining. Presumably patients with a greater ability to perceive and use dynamic components would respond to dynamically oriented therapy by using their ability. By contrast, patients who lack such ability would likely experience more difficulties in therapy. Eventually they might feel that they do not speak the same language and do not fit, and thus become dissatisfied to the point of dropping out. If, in addition, they were symptomatic and experienced a sense of urgency about finding answers to their personal problems, they might be less patient in struggling with the orientation of the therapy group and more prone to leaving. Whereas the available findings are consistent with this conceptualization, one missing element in the current study is a direct measure of the patients' inner struggle with the orientation of therapy. Most dropouts left therapy early (after one or two sessions) before their feelings became evident, and they were not immediately interviewed by the research personnel. Obtaining a direct assessment of the patient's feelings in the sessions, and especially at the time of departure, would be a useful objective for future research.

The relationships between PM and therapy outcome and psychodynamic work and therapy outcome were not strong. A statistical factor that may have contributed to this pattern was the limited range among the scores of the variables. As indicated previously, the correlations were based on remainers, who generally tend to be more satisfied with therapy. In addition, in the case of PM, many of the low-PM patients had dropped out of therapy. Of the 76 remainers, 55 (72.4%) were high-PM patients. Setting this problem aside, there still may be too many other influential events and variables intervening between the initial assessment of PM and the posttherapy assessment of outcome to allow a high correlation. The same may be said for the relationship between work and outcome, as well as the evident limitation of the PWORS in accounting for work only in the form of overt verbal behavior. The identification of other important intervening variables and the use of more inclusive measures of therapy process also represent worthwhile objectives for future research.

Two somewhat different clinical implications follow from the findings concerning the relationships between PM and both working and remaining. The first concerns the process of selecting patients for short-term loss groups. From the data one could conclude that low-PM patients should not be offered a loss group of the type studied. Low-PM patients appear to work less and drop out more frequently. Losing three or four patients in a therapy group of seven is certainly a different clinical experience than losing only one patient. A high dropout rate can have negative repercussions for the entire group. It is possible that a loss group of a different conceptual and technical orientation, one that does *not* focus upon psychodynamic components, would be more suitable for low-PM patients. Or a more structured and/or supportive technique that is less anxiety provoking might be more appropriate.

The second clinical implication concerns the process of preparing patients for short-term loss groups. An examination of the outcome data revealed that some of the low-PM patients did very well. On some measures they did better than high-PM patients. That suggests the possibility that better methods of retaining low-PM patients should be devised. With regard to preparation procedures, the stability findings suggest that it is probably not feasible to attempt to transform a low-PM patient into a high-PM patient. Nevertheless, low-PM patients could be sensitized to a psychodynamic approach and trained to have realistic expectations. Such preparation might help them better endure the difficult initial stage of therapy until bonding with others or the group had occurred. It is possible that low-PM patients represent high-risk, high-gain cases. They are high risk in terms of dropping out prematurely and high gain in terms of therapy outcome if they remain. It is also possible that the low-PM patients who remained and did well were benefiting from what are referred to as nonspecific therapeutic factors, for example, support, that were part of the dynamically oriented loss groups. If so, an alternative approach that emphasized such factors might be more appropriate. This possibility will be considered more fully in the next chapter. Clearly the question is testable, and one or more subsequent studies may reveal the best type of treatment for low-PM patients.

CHAPTER **10**

Conclusions and Future Directions

This book has described an approach to treatment for patients who have not adapted well to the loss of significant persons in their lives. The ubiquitous experience of loss owing to such events as death, separation, and divorce was reaffirmed through a review of the epidemiologic data. Negative experiences associated with loss were also reviewed. The patients who received treatment in the Short-Term Group Therapy Program for Loss Patients were symptomatic, presented themselves to an outpatient department of psychiatry, and were identified by clinician-assessors as people who might benefit from treatment in the program. In other words, they constituted a clinical sample.

The approach to treatment represents one of the unique features highlighted in the book. There are a number of characteristics that serve to distinguish our approach to treatment from others. First, it is a psychosocial form of treatment, in contrast to a biological form such as medication. Second, it is a form of psychotherapy, which means that it focuses more on internal psychological events than on overt behavior. Third, it is psychodynamic in orientation, with a conceptual emphasis on unconscious conflictual components such as wishes, anxiety, and defenses and a technical emphasis on interpretation. Fourth, it is a group form of treatment, thereby involving an entire set of patients in interaction with a therapist, as opposed to a more private, one-to-one relationship between patient and therapist. Fifth, it is a time-limited form of treatment with a predefined beginning and end, as opposed to a form of therapy with an open-ended therapeutic contract. Considering all five of these characteristics, the form of treatment in our program can be summarized as time-limited, short-term, dynamically oriented group psychotherapy.

Other types of intervention for persons suffering from loss that have been described in the literature include some, but not all, of the above five characteristics. For example, the interpretive technique of Raphael's (1983) approach may be regarded as dynamically oriented psychotherapy, although individual in form. Marmar, Horowitz, Weiss, Wilmer, and Kaltreider (1988) also described an individual form of dynamically oriented psychotherapy for persons adjusting to loss. In addition, a variety of time-limited group intervention methods were described in Chapters 3 and 7. Invariably, though, they tended to emphasize support and education, and the participants were usually experiencing normal rather than pathologic reactions to grief. In particular, the combination of interpretive (dynamic) psychotherapy in a time-limited group format with psychiatric outpatients distinguishes the short-term group therapy of our program from other interventions described in the literature.

Before initiating the program we had genuine doubts about the feasibility of the treatment approach. People who have difficulty adjusting to loss are often viewed as overly dependent. Given that the treatment approach does not emphasize the provision of support for individual patients, it was reasonable to question how it would be tolerated by an entire group of relatively "dependent" patients. In addition, the total amount of treatment provided (twelve 90-minute group sessions) appeared to be quite limited for a dynamically oriented form of therapy. There was also reason to question how the patients would tolerate another loss in their lives. In the case of the therapy group, the loss was a multiple one that included other patients and the therapist as well as the group. Although there were theoretical reasons to suggest that the treatment approach ought to be effective, and the results of pilot work with the therapy technique were favorable, the questions required a more substantive type of evidence in order to alleviate our various concerns. The method of providing that evidence represented a second unique feature of the book, namely our controlled, clinical trial outcome study.

As highlighted in Chapter 8, a number of aspects of the clinical trial indicate that its findings should be taken seriously. The study involved a large clinical sample. It included 154 patients, of whom 109 began one of the 16 therapy groups. An examination of diagnoses and initial levels of disturbance on outcome variables revealed that the patients were a genuine clinical sample. The treatment and control conditions were very well balanced on a large number of potentially confounding variables. The therapists were experienced, and the treatment technique was verified by a process analysis of a large number of tape-recorded sessions. A comprehensive battery of outcome measures was used. The results favored treated patients over control patients according to criteria of statistical significance, magnitude of effect, and clinical importance. At follow-up 90% of the patients were reassessed, and the results indicated that the benefits had been maintained or enhanced. Thus the methodology, which exemplified contemporary standards for clinical trial research, and the overall findings provided strong evidence of superior outcome for treated patients as compared with control patients.

A third, relatively unique feature of the book has been the attempt to understand some of the mechanisms underlying the process of therapy by carefully measuring aspects of patient personality and patient performance and examining their association with other clinically relevant variables. Special attention was given to the concept of psychological mindedness because of its apparent theoretical relevance to the psychodynamic orientation of the therapy groups. The clinical trial study provided an opportunity to acquire additional psychometric information about the newly developed measure and to test some hypotheses about how patients work, why they remain or drop out, and the ways in which they benefit from the therapy groups. The significant relationships that were found between psychological mindedness and both working and remaining suggest that it is indeed a theoretically relevant patient characteristic for the therapy groups of the program. An additionally appealing aspect of the measure is its time-efficient quality. By comparison, the measure of psychodynamic work was time-intensive. It served two distinct purposes in the study. First, it provided a means of verifying the nature of the therapy that was actually provided by the therapists. Second, it allowed the examination of relationships between psychological mindedness and work, and between work and therapy outcome. The findings indicated that the former relationship (between psychological mindedness and work) was clearly stronger than the latter.

LIMITATIONS OF THE RESEARCH PROJECT AND QUALIFICATIONS ASSOCIATED WITH THE RESEARCH FINDINGS

Despite the number of strengths inherent in the research methodology of the clinical trial investigation, the evidence is nonetheless based upon a single study. Clearly no single study is without its limitations or potential biases. Therefore the findings must be regarded as tentative and in need of replication in other clinical settings before they can be fully accepted. Several limitations of the research project will be considered next.

One limitation concerns the possibility that the therapy may be suitable for a more restricted patient population than originally anticipated. The immediate treatment condition of the study is probably more comparable to the usual clinic situation than the delay condition, given the 3-month delay associated with the latter. In the immediate treatment condition, 19% of the patients who had agreed to start treatment and who had already completed their initial assessments changed their minds and never began therapy. They were labeled "decliners." On the one hand, because the patients declined before they even started, this form of attrition may be more associated with the nature of loss patients (e.g., highly ambivalent) than with the form of therapy. On the other hand, negative anticipations about joining the particular form of therapy—time-limited, dynamically oriented group therapy—may have been influential. In either case the results suggest that a substantial proportion of selected patients may not start therapy. Of those patients who did start therapy in the immediate condition, about one in three, or 34.5%, terminated prematurely. While this is not a particularly high percentage for group therapy, it is nonetheless substantial, and when combined with the percentage for decliners comprises almost one half of the selected patients. It is possible that a more extensive or different method of preparation might reduce the extent of attrition, but that remains to be demonstrated. Whereas the associations that were found between such patient characteristics as psychological mindedness or initial disturbance and dropping out are informative, they seem more relevant to excluding patients rather than to retaining them. Again, the extent to which patients who are at high risk for dropping out (e.g., disturbed patients of low psychological mindedness) can be retained by means of special pretherapy training or alternative therapy techniques has yet to be determined.

A second limitation of the research project is the absence of an additional treatment condition. If the design had included a second form of treatment, its results could have been compared with our approach to short-term group psychotherapy. Although each form of therapy has certain unique characteristics, some characteristics are shared with other forms of therapy. The shared characteristics are known in the literature as common or nonspecific factors. Such influential figures in the field of individual therapy as Carl Rogers (1957) and Jerome Frank (1973) have emphasized the importance of common factors. Examples include characteristics attributed to patients (e.g., trust), therapists (e.g., empathy), groups (e.g., cohesion), settings (e.g., a clinic), treatments (e.g., a rationale), and patient–therapist relation-ships (e.g., collaborative). Common factors are often viewed as provid-ing support, reassurance, and encouragment. They may bring about a boost in morale, an increased sense of mastery, or a rise in positive expectations. Whereas different forms of therapy may differ consider-ably in format, they may also share a number of common factors.

Some investigators have emphasized the importance of common factors over those considered to be unique to a particular form of therapy. Comparative outcome studies that have found significant changes from before to after therapy for each of the treatments, but nonsignificant differences between the treatments, have been regarded as providing evidence of the impact of common factors. With regard to the present study the question is "To what extent were the benefits associated with the therapy groups in the program due to common factors?" Stated somewhat differently, "To what extent might any new form of therapy that provides support and boosts morale bring about multiple benefits?" In the present study the inclusion of a second form of treatment that differed on unique factors (e.g., one that minimized the use of interpretation) but shared common factors (e.g., therapist empathy and a convincing rationale) would have provided an oppor-tunity to compare the relative importance of the two kinds of factors.

Independent of the distinction between common and unique fac-tors is the concept of therapeutic factors. In the group therapy litera-ture they have often been referred to as curative factors. Therapeutic (curative) factors are those variables that are regarded as responsible for therapeutic change. One of the first attempts to delineate such variables for group therapy was made by Corsini and Rosenberg (1955), who identified nine different factors. Later these variables were modified and expanded upon by Irvin Yalom in his well-known text concerning the theory and practice of group psychotherapy (Yalom, 1985). They have also been the focus of a book by Bloch and Crouch (1985).

Whether a particular therapeutic factor is regarded as common or unique depends on the different therapies that are being compared. Some of the factors that have received the most attention are those that are regarded as unique to group therapy as compared with individual therapy, but common among different group therapies. Examples include universality (a sense of shared experience), altruism (helping one another), and cohesion (bonds among the members of the group). Each requires the presence of a set of peers, that is, other patients. As MacKenzie (1990) has pointed out, the presence of group members provides unique opportunities for such additional therapeutic factors as modeling, vicarious learning, guidance, and education to occur as well. There is little doubt in our minds that patients in the loss group program benefited from the presence of other patients in the therapy groups and that a number of therapeutic factors contributed to the favorable outcomes that were observed. The relative contribution of the different therapeutic factors, including insight into long-standing conflicts involving loss, which we have emphasized in our conceptual and technical approach, is not possible to determine from our present research project. It is an issue that is definitely worthy of future investigation.

In future research a form of therapy that would provide a useful comparison condition for our approach to treatment studies is supportive group therapy. In the last few years several books (Rockland, 1989; Werman, 1984) and reviews (Winston, Pinsker, & McCullough, 1986) have focused on psychodynamically oriented, supportive therapy. Although there appears to be no standard definition for supportive therapy, a number of features are commonly emphasized. Its objective is to improve immediate adaptation to the patient's current life situation, rather than to enhance insight about conflicts. Supportive therapy focuses on conscious processes, reality, and current relationships with people outside the session (rather than unconscious processes, fantasy, and early relationships or the patient–therapist relationship). In response to the patient's efforts, it offers praise, not scrutiny, and attempts to minimize, rather than accentuate, anxiety and regression in the therapy sessions. Overall, it provides more immediate gratification to the patient. Rockland argues that, contrary to popular belief, supportive therapy is characterized by specific technical features that require training and that should be a part of each therapist's repertoire.

Few studies have attempted to evaluate or compare the effectiveness of supportive psychotherapy against that of other forms of psychotherapy. In a study with phobic patients that compared supportive individual psychotherapy plus imipramine with behavior therapy plus imipramine, there were no significant differences between the two treatments and each was associated with favorable results (Klein, Zitrin, Woerner, & Ross, 1983; Zitrin, Klein, & Woerner, 1978). In a study with chronic obstructive pulmonary disease patients, supportive individual psychotherapy equaled or exceeded the results of analytic (interpretive) psychotherapy (Rosser, Denford, Heslop, Kinston, Machlin, Minty, Moynihan, Muir, Rein, & Guz, 1983). Supportive psychotherapy was also one of the treatments in the Menninger Psychotherapy Research Project, where it was compared with expressive (interpretive) psychotherapy and psychoanalysis. In a recent overview of the project, Wallerstein (1989) concluded that supportive mechanisms permeated all three types of therapy and accounted for stable and enduring changes. Thus, although the number of studies is small, supportive psychotherapy has made a respectable showing and has exceeded the initial expectations of its investigators.

Those who have reviewed the literature argue that supportive psychotherapy is a highly prevalent form of treatment that has incorrectly been regarded as inferior to interpretive psychotherapy. In his book Rockland (1989) provided two additional conclusions.

> Supportive therapy is probably more effective for less healthy, poorly motivated patients, exploratory therapy for healthier, better motivated patients. Supportive therapy deserves more study, particularly of its outcomes, when applied to patients across the diagnostic spectrum who have varying motivations, degrees of psychological mindedness, and so on. (pp. 242–243)

These conclusions raise the possibility that certain types of patients might do better with a supportive, rather than an interpretive, form of therapy. With regard to the type of patients treated in our program, it is possible that those who are of particularly low psychological mindedness might better tolerate a supportive approach and be less likely to drop out prematurely. It is also possible that they might experience more favorable treatment outcome.

The prospect of finding optimal treatment matches for patients has been an aspiration of psychotherapists and psychotherapy researchers for a number of years. In 1967 Gordon Paul made his often quoted statement about the need to elucidate the relationships among patient, problem, therapist, therapy, and circumstance variables. In the last several years this multivariate approach to understanding the effects of therapy and prescribing the most appropriate form has been the theme of two recent books (Beutler & Clarkin, 1990; Frances, Clarkin, & Perry, 1984) as well as the 1989 three-volume report of the American Psychiatric Association Task Force on Treatment of Psychiatric disorders. A recent special section of the *Journal of Consulting and Clinical Psychology* (1991, April) also focused on the topic of the optimal matching of patients and psychotherapies. Future research investigating patient characteristics such as psychological mindedness with different forms of therapy for patients suffering from loss would certainly contribute relevant information to the field.

There are always limits to the resources available in clinical and research settings. Consequently choices must be made concerning which questions will be addressed during certain periods of time. As indicated in Chapter 7, we were interested in using methodology that would allow us to detect important relationships among the variables at statistical levels of significance. To accomplish that objective, a large sample was required. Thus we decided to concentrate on just one form of therapy and a control condition. As indicated above, over a 4-year period the study involved 154 patients, of whom 109 participated in 16 therapy groups. The sample size allowed for the detection of a number of significant effects that concerned patient attrition, therapy process, and therapy outcome.

With regard to the treatment versus control group outcome findings of the present study, we suspect that some of the unique aspects of the dynamically oriented, group therapy technique were responsible for the greater benefits for treated patients. Consistent interpretive focusing on conflictual components associated with loss in a time-limited group situation is to us a theoretically sound approach to the treatment of loss patients. Thus we believe that the benefits associated with the groups were not entirely due to common factors. We acknowledge, however, that the present study does not allow that issue to be settled. There is little doubt that it is a worthwhile issue, one that we hope to address in subsequent research. However, even if future research were to reveal that the benefits associated with the therapy groups of our program were more a function of common rather than unique factors, we believe that the results of the present study would remain worthwhile. The study has demonstrated the effectiveness of an economical form of therapy for a specific patient population. For that reason the study should encourage others to investigate time-limited, group therapy approaches to the treatment of loss patients.

Some qualifications regarding the findings of the study should also be remembered. As pointed out in Chapter 8, most of the outcome variables significantly favored the treatment condition. However, several of the variables did not change significantly over the course of therapy. The more intractable variables involved interpersonal functioning and dependency. These findings highlight the point that the short-term loss groups should not be viewed as a cure-all. Long-standing interpersonal patterns are not easy to change, certainly not in a matter of a few months. In our opinion it would be theoretically and technically inappropriate to even attempt to change basic character and personality disorders in short-term groups. This would inevitably deflect the therapist and patients from the task at hand. Other forms of treatment that are designed to deal with interpersonal patterns over longer periods of time, for example, long-term group psychotherapy, would be required. Conducting time-limited loss groups for a longer period, such as 6 months or a year, is also a possibility. When longer forms of treatment are considered, the issue of gains versus costs becomes salient. A number of worthwhile gains that were maintained at 6-month follow-up were associated with the 3-month therapy groups of the loss group program. They covered a number of different areas, including the specific target objectives of the patient. The decision to extend the duration of therapy in the hope of effecting additional improvements in interpersonal areas requires the commitment of the primary parties (patient, therapist) and frequently third-party payment sources.

One additional limitation associated with conducting short-term loss groups is the skill required of the therapist. After completing over 25 such groups, we are convinced that loss groups are not for beginners. In Chapter 5 we highlighted many of the demands that are part of the therapist's role. Besides attempting to fulfill such technical criteria as passive encouragement of regression, maintenance of neutrality, analysis of transference, and use of interpretation as a main technique, the therapist is required to consistently focus on the commonalities of the patients and use the structural limitations of the group productively. Typically this involves making frequent interventions, including group-level interpretations. Thus the role demanded of the therapist is an energy-consuming one that requires clinical expertise. At times this role can be quite stressful. The subject matter of these groups, that is, loss, should not be underestimated in terms of its impact on the therapist. Our own experience suggests that ongoing support for loss group therapists in the form of supervision, consultation, or, ideally, an integrated training program is highly recommended.

To repeat what has been stated earlier in this book, we believe that loss groups portray definite patterns that make sense both conceptually and clinically. Learning to recognize the patterns and provide appropriate interventions distinguishes the skillful therapist from the nonskillful. We think that these can be more successfully accomplished if the therapist has had some previous experience with another form of group therapy, for example, dynamically oriented long-term group psychotherapy. Once one has gained experience with short-term loss groups, we believe that the modality can represent a stimulating and rewarding part of one's clinical practice.

In conclusion, we believe that we have identified a viable and cost-effective form of treatment for a prevalent group of psychiatric patients. By the standards of many practitioners, even those of contemporary psychoanalysts, our approach may seem particularly classical or traditional in orientation. As indicated earlier, we were interested in whether adherence to a psychodynamic orientation under the appropriate conditions would be effective with loss patients. The results of our program suggest that time-limited group approaches can be successful if they are specifically tailored to the needs of particular types of patients. Nevertheless, a variety of questions, both theoretical and clinical, remain to be answered. They include such topics as the nature of the therapeutic mechanisms of the treatment, the nature of the patients best suited to the treatment, and comparisons of the results with those of other treatment approaches. Many of the questions that remain to be answered arose from the ongoing collaborative interactions between clinicians and researchers involved in the program and research project, which were rewarding indeed. We hope to discover some of the answers in our future work. We also hope that this book will encourage others to do the same.

References

Alexander, D. A. (1988). Bereavement and the management of grief. *British Journal of Psychiatry, 153,* 860–864.

Alexander, F., & French, T. (1946). *Psychoanalytic therapy: Principles and applications.* New York: Ronald Press.

American Psychiatric Association. (1980). *Diagnostic and statistical manual of mental disorders* (3rd ed.). Washington, DC: Author.

American Psychiatric Association. (1987). *Diagnostic and statistical manual of mental disorders* (3rd ed., rev.). Washington, DC: Author.

American Psychiatric Association Commission on Psychotherapies. (1982). *Psychotherapy research: Methodological and efficacy issues.* Washington, DC: American Psychiatric Association.

American Psychiatric Association Task Force on Treatment of Psychiatric Disorders. (1989). *Treatment of psychiatric disorders.* Washington, DC: American Psychiatric Association.

Ammons, R. B., & Ammons, C. H. (1962). *The Quick Test: Provisional manual.* Missoula, MT: Psychological Test Specialists.

Appelbaum, S. A. (1973). Psychological mindedness: Word, concept, and essence. *International Journal of Psycho-Analysis, 54,* 35–46.

Ariès, P. (1982). *The hour of our death.* New York: Vintage Books.

Ariès, P. (1985). *Images of man and death.* Cambridge, MA: Harvard University Press.

Arthur, B., & Kemme, M. L. (1964). Bereavement in childhood. *Journal of Child Psychology and Psychiatry, 5,* 37–49.

Baekeland, F., & Lundwall, L. (1975). Dropping out of treatment: A critical review. *Psychological Bulletin, 82,* 738–783.

Bagby, R. M., Taylor, G. J., & Ryan, D. (1986). Toronto alexithymia scale: Relationship with personality and psychopathology measures. *Psychotherapy and Psychosomatics, 45,* 207–215.

Barrett, C. J. (1978). Effectiveness of widows' groups in facilitating change. *Journal of Consulting and Clinical Psychology, 46,* 20–31.

Beck, A. P. (1974). Phases in the development of structure in therapy and encounter groups. In D. A. Wexler & L. N. Rice (Eds.), *Innovations in client-centered therapy* (pp. 421–463). New York: Wiley.

Beck, A. T. (1976). *Cognitive therapy and the emotional disorders.* New York: International Universities Press.

Beck, A. T., & Steer, R. A. (1987). *Beck Depression Inventory manual.* New York: Harcourt Brace Jovanovich.

Benedek, E. P. (1984). The impact of parental divorce on children and adolescents. In J. H. Gold (Ed.), *Divorce as a developmental process* (pp. 117–134). Washington, DC: American Psychiatric Press.

Beutler, L. E., & Clarkin, J. F. (1990). *Systematic treatment selection: Toward targeted therapeutic interventions.* New York: Brunner/Mazel.

Bibring, E. (1954). Psychoanalysis and the dynamic psychotherapies. *Journal of the American Psychoanalytic Association, 2,* 745–770.

Bienvenu, J. P., Piper, W. E., Debbane, E. G., & de Carufel, F. L. (1986). On the concept of psychoanalytic work. *American Journal of Psychotherapy, 40,* 277–289.

Bion, W. R. (1959). *Experiences in groups.* New York: Basic Books.

Bloch, I., Roth, J. (Producers), & Cain, C. (Director). (1984). *Stone Boy* [Film]. Beverly Hills, CA: Twentieth Century Fox.

Bloch, S., & Crouch, E. (1985). *Therapeutic factors in group psychotherapy.* Oxford: Oxford University Press.

Bloom-Feshbach, J., Bloom-Feshbach, S., & Associates (Eds.). (1987). *The psychology of separation and loss.* San Francisco: Jossey-Bass.

Bornstein, P. E., Clayton, P. J., Halikas, J. A., Maurice, W. L., & Robins, E. (1973). The depression of widowhood after thirteen months. *British Journal of Psychiatry, 122,* 561–566.

Bowlby, J. (1960). Grief and mourning in infancy and early childhood. *Psychoanalytic Study of the Child, 15,* 9–52.

Bowlby, J. (1963). Pathological mourning and childhood mourning. *Journal of the American Psychoanalytic Association, 11,* 500–541.

Bowlby, J. (1980). *Attachment and loss.* London: Hogarth Press.

Bruch, B. (1989). Mourning and failure to mourn. *Contemporary Psychoanalysis, 25,* 608–623.

Budman, S. H., Bennett, M. J., & Wisneski, M. J. (1981). An adult developmental model of short-term group psychotherapy. In S. H. Budman (Ed.), *Forms of brief therapy* (pp. 305–342). New York: Guilford Press.

Budman, S. H., Clifford, M., Bader, L., & Bader, B. (1981). Experiential pre-group preparation and screening. *Group, 5,* 19–26.

Budman, S. H., Demby, A., Feldstein, M., & Gold, M. (1984). The effects of time-limited group psychotherapy: A controlled study. *International Journal of Group Psychotherapy, 34,* 587–603.

Budman, S. H., Demby, A., & Randall, M. (1980). Short-term group psychotherapy: Who succeeds, who fails? *Group, 4,* 3–16.

Budman, S. H., Randall, M., & Demby, A. (1981). Outcome in short-term group psychotherapy. *Group, 5,* 37–51.

Call, J., & Wolfenstein, M. (1976). Effects on adults of object loss in the first five years. *Journal of the American Psychoanalytic Association, 24,* 659–668.

Campbell, D. T., & Stanley, J. C. (1963). *Experimental and quasi-experimental designs for research.* Chicago: Rand McNally College Publishing.

Chapman, A. (1959). The concept of nemesis in psychoneurosis. *The Journal of Nervous and Mental Disease, 129,* 29–34.

Clayton, P. J. (1973). The clinical morbidity of the first year of bereavement: A review. *Comprehensive Psychiatry, 14,* 151–157.

Clayton, P. J., Herjanic, M., & Murphy, G. (1972). Mourning and depression: Their similarities and differences. *Canadian Journal of Psychiatry, 19,* 309–312.

Conte, H. R., Plutchik, R., Jung, B. B., Picard, S., Karaso, T. B., & Lotterman, A. (1990). Psychological mindedness as a predictor of psychotherapy outcome: A preliminary report. *Comprehensive Psychiatry, 31,* 426–431.

Cooper, A. M. (1987). Changes in psychoanalytic ideas: Transference interpretation. *Journal of the American Psychoanalytic Association, 35,* 77–98.

Corsini, R., & Rosenberg, B. (1955). Mechanisms of group psychotherapy: Processes and dynamics. *Journal of Abnormal and Social Psychology, 51,* 406–411.

Davanloo, H. (Ed.). (1978). *Basic principles and techniques in short-term dynamic psychotherapy.* New York: Spectrum.

Derogatis, L. R. (1977). *SCL-90 administration, scoring and procedures manual: 1.* Baltimore, MD: Johns Hopkins University Press.

Dietrich, D. R. (1989). Early childhood parent death, psychic trauma and organization, and object relations. In D. R. Dietrich & P. Shabad (Eds.), *The problem of loss and mourning: Psychoanalytic perspectives* (pp. 289–290). Madison, CT: International Universities Press.

Dietrich, D. R., & Shabad, P. (Eds.). (1990). *The problem of loss and mourning: Psychoanalytic perspectives.* Madison, CT: International Universities Press.

Ehrenreich, J. H. (1989). Transference: One concept or many? *Psychoanalytic Review, 76,* 37–65.

Fenichel, O. (1945). *The psychoanalytic theory of neurosis.* New York: W.W. Norton.

Fenichel, O. (1953). Specific forms of the Oedipus complex. In H. Fenichel & D. Rapaport (Eds.), *The collected papers of Otto Fenichel* (pp. 203–220). New York: W. W. Norton.

Ferenczi, S., & Rank, O. (1925). *The development of psychoanalysis.* New York: Nervous and Mental Disease Publication Company.

Frances, A., Clarkin, J., & Perry, S. (1984). *Differential therapeutics in psychiatry: The art and science of treatment selection.* New York: Brunner/Mazel.

Frank, J. D. (1973). *Persuasion and healing: A comparative study of psychotherapy.* Baltimore, MD: Johns Hopkins University Press.

Freud, S. (1957a). Mourning and melancholia. In J. Strachey (Ed. and Trans.), *The standard edition of the complete psychological works of Sigmund Freud* (Vol. 14, pp. 239–260). London: Hogarth Press. (Original work published 1917)

Freud, S. (1957b). On narcissism: An introduction. In J. Strachey (Ed. and Trans.), *The standard edition of the complete psychological works of Sigmund Freud* (Vol. 14, pp. 69–102). London: Hogarth Press. (Original work published 1914)

Freud, S. (1957c). Thoughts for the times on war and death—II. Our attitude towards death. In J. Strachey (Ed. and Trans.), *The standard edition of the complete psychological works of Sigmund Freud* (Vol. 14, pp. 289–300). London: Hogarth Press. (Original work published 1915)

Freud, S. (1963). Introductory lectures on psychoanalysis. In J. Strachey (Ed. and Trans.), *The standard edition of the complete psychological works of Sigmund Freud* (Vols. 15–16). London: Hogarth Press. (Original work published 1916–1917)

Freud, S. (1964). Constructions in analysis. In J. Strachey (Ed. and Trans.), *The standard edition of the complete psychological works of Sigmund Freud* (Vol. 23, pp. 257–269). London: Hogarth Press. (Original work published 1937)

Furman, E. (1974). *A child's parent dies: Studies in childhood bereavement.* New Haven, CT: Yale University Press.

Garfield, S. L., & Bergin, A. E. (Eds.). (1986). *Handbook of psychotherapy and behavior change* (3rd ed.). New York: Wiley.

Gay, P. (1988). *Freud: A life for our time.* New York: W. W. Norton.

Gill, M. M. (1954). Psychoanalysis and exploratory psychotherapy. *Journal of the American Psychoanalytic Association, 2,* 771–797.

Gill, M. M. (1984). Psychoanalysis and psychotherapy: A revision. *International Review of Psychoanalysis, 11,* 161–179.

Goldberg, D. A., Schuyler, W. R., Bransfield, D., & Savino, P. (1983). Focal group psychotherapy: A dynamic approach. *International Journal of Group Psychotherapy, 33,* 413–431.

Gorer, G. (1965). *Death, grief and mourning in contemporary Britain.* Garden City, NJ: Doubleday.

Gough, H. G. (1957). *California Psychological Inventory.* Palo Alto, CA: Consulting Psychological Press.

Greenson, R. R. (1967). *The technique and practice of psychoanalysis.* New York: International Universities Press.

Hilgard, J. R. (1969). Depressive and psychotic states as anniversaries to sibling death in childhood. In E. S. Shneidman & M. J. Ortega (Eds.), *Aspects of depression* (pp. 197–211). Boston: Little, Brown.

Hill, W. F. (1965). *Hill Interaction Matrix.* Los Angeles: University of California, Youth Study Center.

Hirschfeld, R. M. A., Klerman, G., Gough, H., Barrett, J., Korchin, S., & Chodoff, P. (1977). A measure of interpersonal dependency. *Journal of Personality Assessment, 41,* 610–618.

Holmes, T. H., & Rahe, R. H. (1967). The social readjustment rating scale. *Journal of Psychosomatic Research, 11,* 213–218.

Horowitz, L. (1989, June). *People who describe other people clearly are better candidates for brief dynamic psychotherapy.* Paper presented at the 20th Annual Meeting of the Society for Psychotherapy Research, Toronto, Ontario, Canada.

Horowitz, M. J. (1990). A model of mourning: Change in schemas of self and other. *Journal of the American Psychoanalytic Association, 38,* 297–324.

Horowitz, M. J., Marmar, C., Weiss, D. S., DeWitt, K. N., & Rosenbaum, R. (1984). Brief psychotherapy of bereavement reactions. *Archives of General Psychiatry, 41,* 438–448.

Horowitz, M. J., Wilner, N., & Alvarez, W. (1979). Impact of event scale: A measure of subjective stress. *Psychosomatic Medicine, 41,* 209–218.

Horowitz, M. J., Wilner, N., Marmar, C., & Krupnick, J. (1980). Pathological grief and the activation of latent self-images. *The American Journal of Psychiatry, 137,* 1157–1162.

Hudson, W. W., Thyer, B. A., & Stocks, J. T. (1985). Assessing the importance of experimental outcomes. *Journal of Social Service Research, 8,* 87–98.

Imber, S. D., Lewis, P. M., & Loiselle, R. H. (1979). Uses and abuses of the brief intervention group. *International Journal of Group Psychotherapy, 29,* 39–49.

Jackson, D. M. (1974). *Personality Research Form manual.* Goshen, NY: Research Psychologist's Press.

Jacobs, S., & Kim, K. (1990). Psychiatric complications of bereavement. *Psychiatric Annals, 20,* 314–317.

Jacobson, N. S., & Revenstorf, D. (1988). Statistics for assessing the clinical significance of psychotherapy techniques: Issues, problems, and new developments. *Behavioral Assessment, 10,* 133–145.

Kaul, T. J., & Bednar, R. L. (1986). Experiential group research: Results, questions and suggestions. In S. L. Garfield & A. E. Bergin (Eds.), *Handbook for psychotherapy and behavior change* (3rd ed., pp. 671–714). New York: Wiley.

Kernberg, O., Burstein, E., Coyne, L., Appelbaum, H., Horowitz, L., & Voth, H. (1972). Psychotherapy and psychoanalysis: Final report of the Menninger Foundation's psychotherapy research project. *Bulletin of the Menninger Clinic, 36,* 1–275.

Kirkpatrick, M. (1984). Some clinical perceptions of middle-aged divorcing women. In J. H. Gold (Ed.), *Divorce as a developmental process* (pp. 81–99). Washington, DC: American Psychiatric Press.

Klein, D. F., Zitrin, C. M., Woerner, M., & Ross, D. (1983). Treatment of phobias. *Archives of General Psychiatry, 40,* 139–145.

Klein, M. (1948). *Contributions to psychoanalysis 1921–1945.* London: Hogarth Press.

Klein, R. H. (1985). Some principles of short-term group therapy. *International Journal of Group Psychotherapy, 35,* 309–330.

Klerman, G. L., Weissman, M. M., Rounsaville, B. J., & Chevron, E. S. (1984). *Interpersonal psychotherapy of depression.* New York: Basic Books.

Krupnick, J. L., & Solomon, F. (1987). Death of a parent or sibling during childhood. In J. Bloom-Feshback, S. Bloom-Feshback, & Associates (Eds.), *The psychology of separation and loss* (pp. 345–371). San Francisco: Jossey-Bass.

Lambert, M. J., Shapiro, D. A., & Bergin, A. E. (1986). The effectiveness of psychotherapy. In S. L. Garfield & A. E. Bergin (Eds.), *Handbook of Psychotherapy and Behavior Change* (3rd ed., pp. 157–211). New York: Wiley.

Laplanche, J., & Pontalis, J. B. (1973). *The language of psychoanalysis* (D. Nicholson-Smith, Trans.). New York: W.W. Norton. (Original work published 1967)

Lapointe, K. A., & Rimm, D. C. (1980). Cognitive, assertive, and insight-oriented group therapies in treatment of reactive depression in women. *Psychotherapy: Theory, Research, and Practice, 17,* 312–321.

Lazare, A. (1989). Bereavement and unresolved grief. In A. Lazare (Ed.), *Outpatient psychiatry: Diagnosis and treatment* (pp. 381–397). Baltimore, MD: Williams & Wilkins.

Lerner, H. D., & Lerner, P. M. (1987). Separation, depression, and object loss: Indications for narcissism and object relations. In J. Bloom-Feshback, S. Bloom-Feshback, & Associates (Eds.), *The psychology of separation and loss* (pp. 375–395). San Francisco: Jossey-Bass.

Lewinsohn, P. M. (1973). Clinical and theoretical aspects of depression. In K. S. Calhoun, H. E. Adams, & K. M. Mitchell (Eds.), *Innovative treatment in psychopathology* (pp. 63–120). New York: Wiley.

Lieberman, M. A., & Videka-Sherman, L. (1986). The impact of self-help groups on the mental health of widows and widowers. *American Journal of Orthopsychiatry, 56,* 435–449.

Lindemann, E. (1944). Symptomatology and management of acute grief. *American Journal of Psychiatry, 101,* 141–148.

Loewenstein, R. M. (1951). The problem of interpretation. *Psychoanalytic Quarterly, 20,* 1–14.

Lohr, R., & Chethik, M. (1990). Parental loss through divorce: Dimensions for the loss experience. In D. R. Dietrich & P. Shabad (Eds.), *The problem of loss and mourning: Psychoanalytic perspectives* (pp. 239–242). Madison, CT: International Universities Press.

Lothstein, L. M. (1978). The group psychotherapy dropout phenomenon revisited. *American Journal of Psychiatry, 135,* 1492–1495.

MacKenzie, K. R. (1990). *Time-limited group psychotherapy.* Washington, DC: American Psychiatric Press.

MacKenzie, K. R., & Livesley, W. J. (1983). A developmental model for brief group therapy. In R. R. Dies & K. R. MacKenzie (Eds.), *Advances in group psychotherapy: Integrating research and practice* (pp. 101–116). New York: International Universities Press.

Malan, D. H. (1976). *The frontier of brief psychotherapy.* New York: Plenum.

Mann, J. (1973). *Time-limited psychotherapy.* Cambridge, MA: Harvard University Press.

Marmar, C. R., Horowitz, M. J., Weiss, D. S., Wilner, N. R., & Kaltreider, N. B. (1988). A controlled trial of brief psychotherapy and mutual-help group treatment of conjugal bereavement. *American Journal of Psychiatry, 145,* 203–209.

McCallum, M., & Piper, W. E. (1988). Psychoanalytically oriented short-term groups for outpatients: Unsettled issues. *Group, 12,* 21–32.

McCallum, M., & Piper, W. E. (1990). The psychological mindedness assessment procedure. *Psychological Assessment: A Journal of Consulting and Clinical Psychology, 2,* 412–418.

McCallum, M., & Piper, W. E. (in press). Dropping out from short-term group therapy. *Psychotherapy.*

Melges, F. T., & DeMaso, D. R. (1980). Grief-resolution therapy: Reliving, revising, and revisiting. *American Journal of Psychotherapy, 34,* 51–61.

Osterweis, M., Solomon, F., & Green, M. (1984). Bereavement: Reactions, consequences and care. *A report of the Institute of Medicine, National Academy of Sciences.* Washington, DC: National Academy Press.

Parkes, C. M. (1972). *Bereavement studies of grief in adult life.* New York: International Universities Press.

Parkes, C. M. (1990). Risk factors in bereavement: Implications for the prevention and treatment of pathologic grief. *Psychiatric Annals, 20,* 308–313.

Paul, G. L. (1967). Outcome research in psychotherapy. *Journal of Consulting Psychology, 31,* 109–118.

Piper, W. E. (1988). Psychotherapy research in the 1980s: Defining areas of consensus and controversy. *Hospital and Community Psychiatry, 39,* 1055–1063.

Piper, W. E., Debbane, E. G., Bienvenu, J. P., & Garant, J. (1982). A study of group pretraining for group psychotherapy. *International Journal of Group Psychotherapy, 32,* 309–325.

Piper, W. E., Debbane, E. G., Bienvenu, J. P., & Garant, J. (1984). A comparative study of four forms of psychotherapy. *Journal of Consulting and Clinical Psychology, 52,* 268–279.

Piper, W. E., Debbane, E. G., de Carufel, F. L., & Bienvenu, J. P. (1987). A system for differentiating therapist interpretations and other interventions. *Bulletin of the Menninger Clinic, 51,* 532–550.

Piper, W. E., Debbane, E. G., & Garant, J. (1977). An outcome study of group therapy. *Archives of General Psychiatry, 34,* 1027–1032.

Piper, W. E., de Carufel, F. L., & Szkrumelak, N. (1985). Patient predictors of process and outcome in short-term individual psychotherapy. *Journal of Nervous and Mental Disease, 173,* 726–733.

Piper, W. E., Marrache, M., Lacroix, R., Richardsen, A. M., & Jones, B. D. (1983). Cohesion as a basic bond in groups. *Human Relations, 36,* 93–108.

Piper, W. E., & McCallum, M. (1989). Psychodynamische arbeit als ein wirkfaktor in der gruppenpsychotherapie. In V. Tschuschke & D. Czogalik (Hrsg.), *Psychotherapie—Welche effekte verändern?* (pp. 349–368). Heidelberg: Springer-Verlag.

Piper, W. E., & McCallum, M. (in press). Psychodynamic work and object rating system. In A. P. Beck, L. R. Green, & C. M. Lewis (Eds.), *Process in therapeutic groups: A handbook of systems of analysis.* New York: Guilford Press.

Piper, W. E., & Perrault, E. L. (1989). Pretherapy preparation for group members. *International Journal of Group Psychotherapy, 39,* 17–34.

Poey, K. (1985). Guidelines for the practice of brief, dynamic group therapy. *International Journal of Group Psychotherapy, 35,* 331–354.

Pollock, G. (1989). *The mourning-liberation process* (Vols. 1–2). Madison, CT: International Universities Press.

Pynoos, R. S., & Nader, K. (1990). Children's exposure to violence and traumatic death. *Psychiatric Annals, 20,* 334–344.

Ramsey, R. W. (1977). Behavioral approaches to bereavement. *Behavioral Research and Therapy, 15*, 131–140.

Raphael, B. (1983). *The anatomy of bereavement*. New York: Basic Books.

Raphael, B., & Middleton, W. (1987). Current state of research in the field of bereavement. *Israel Journal of Psychiatry and Related Sciences, 24*, 5–32.

Raphael, B., & Middleton, W. (1990). What is pathologic grief? *Psychiatric Annals, 20*, 304–307.

Rockland, L. H. (1989). *Supportive therapy: A psychodynamic approach*. New York: Basic Books.

Rogers, C. (1957). The necessary and sufficient conditions of therapeutic personality change. *Journal of Consulting and Clinical Psychology, 21*, 95–103.

Rogers, J., Vachon, M. L. S., Lyall, W. A., Sheldon, A., & Freeman, S. J. J. (1980). A self-help program for widows as an independent community service. *Hospital and Community Psychiatry, 31*, 845–847.

Rosen, V. H. (1977). The nature of verbal interventions in psychoanalysis. In S. Atkin & M. E. Jucovy (Eds.), *Style, character and language* (pp. 219–239). New York: Jason Aronson.

Rosenbaum, R. L., & Horowitz, M. J. (1983). Motivation for psychotherapy: A factorial and conceptual analysis. *Psychological Theory, Research, and Practice, 20*, 346–354.

Rosenberg, M. (1979). *Conceiving the self*. New York: Basic Books.

Rosser, R., Denford, J., Heslop, A., Kinston, W., Machlin, D., Minty, K., Moynihan, C., Muir, B., Rein, L., & Guz, A. (1983). Breathlessness and psychiatric morbidity in chronic bronchitis and emphysema: A study of psychotherapeutic management. *Psychological Medicine, 13*, 93–110.

Rubin, S. S. (1984). Mourning distinct from melancholia: The resolution of bereavement. *British Journal of Medical Psychology, 57*, 339–345.

Rycroft, C. (1958). An enquiry into the function of words in the psychoanalytical situation. *International Journal of Psychoanalysis, 39*, 408–415.

Sandler, J., Dare, C., & Holder, A. (1970). Basic psychoanalytic concepts: III. Transference. *British Journal of Psychiatry, 116*, 667–672.

Schuchter, S. R., & Zisook, S. (1987). The therapeutic tasks of grief. In S. Zisook (Ed.), *Biopsychosocial aspects of bereavement* (pp. 177–189). Washington, DC: American Psychiatric Press.

Schwary, R. L. (Producer), & Redford, R. (Director). (1980). *Ordinary People* [Film]. Los Angeles, CA: Paramount-Wildwood Pictures.

Sifneos, P. E. (1979). *Short-term dynamic psychotherapy evaluation and technique*. New York: Plenum.

Sifneos, P. E. (1981). Short-term anxiety-provoking psychotherapy: Its history, technique, outcome, and instruction. In S. H. Budman (Ed.), *Forms of brief therapy* (pp. 45–81). New York: Guilford Press.

Shackleton, C. H. (1984). The psychology of grief: A review. *Advances in Behaviour Research and Therapy, 6*, 153–205.

Silverman, P. R. (1969). The widow-to-widow program: An experiment in preventive intervention. *Mental Hygiene, 53*, 333–337.

Smith, M. H., Glass, G. V., & Miller, T. I. (1980). *The benefits of psychotherapy.* Baltimore, MD: Johns Hopkins University Press.

Statistics Canada. (1981). *Census 1981: Total income* (Catalogue 92-928). Ottawa: Canadian Government Publishing Center.

Statistics Canada. (1986). *Census 1986: Age, sex and marital status* (Catalogue 93-101). Ottawa: Canadian Government Publishing Center.

Stiles, W. B. (1988). Psychotherapy process-outcome correlations may be misleading. *Psychotherapy, 25,* 27–35.

Stroebe, W., & Stroebe, M. S. (1987). *Bereavement and health: The psychological and physical consequences of partner loss.* Cambridge: Cambridge University Press.

Tahka, V. (1984). Dealing with object loss. *Scandinavian Psychoanalytic Review, 7,* 13–33.

Thelen, H. A., Stock, D., Hill, W. F., Ben-Zeev, S., & Heintz, I. (1954). *Methods for studying work and emotionality in group operation.* Chicago: University of Chicago, Human Dynamics Laboratory.

Tolor, A., & Reznikoff, M. (1960). A new approach to insight: A preliminary report. *Journal of Nervous and Mental Disease, 130,* 286–296.

Toseland, R. W., & Siporin, M. (1986). When to recommend group treatment: A review of the clinical and group literature. *International Journal of Group Psychotherapy, 36,* 171–201.

Tyson, R. L. (1983). Some narcissistic consequences of object loss: A developmental view. *Psychoanalytic Quarterly, 52,* 205–224.

U.S. Bureau of the Census. (1978). *Statistical abstract of the United States: 1978* (99th ed.). Washington, DC: U.S. Government Printing Office.

U.S. Department of Justice. (1985). *Crime in the United States.* Washington, DC: Author.

Vachon, M. L. S., Lyall, W. A. L., Rogers, J., Freedman-Letofsky, K., & Freeman, S. J. J. (1980). A controlled study of self-help intervention for widows. *American Journal of Psychiatry, 137,* 1380–1384.

Volkan, V. D. (1975). "Re-grief" therapy. In B. Schoenberg & I. Gerber (Eds.), *Bereavement: Its psychological aspects* (pp. 334–350). New York: Columbia University Press.

Wallerstein, J. S. (1986). Women after divorce: Preliminary report from a ten-year follow-up. *American Journal of Orthopsychiatry, 56,* 65–77.

Wallerstein, R. S. (1989). The psychotherapy research project of the Menninger Foundation: An overview. *Journal of Consulting and Clinical Psychology, 57,* 195–205.

Walls, N., & Meyers, A. W. (1985). Outcome in group treatment for bereavement: Experimental results and recommendations for clinical practice. *International Journal of Mental Health, 13,* 126–147.

Waskow, I. E., & Parloff, M. B. (1975). *Psychotherapy change measures.* Washington, DC: U.S. Government Printing Office.

Weissman, M. M., Paykel, E. S., Siegel, R., & Klerman, G. L. (1971). The social role performance of depressed women: A comparison with a normal sample. *American Journal of Orthopsychiatry, 41,* 390–405.

Weitzman, L. (1985). *The Divorce Revolution*. New York: Free Press.

Werman, D. S. (1984). *The practice of supportive psychotherapy*. New York: Brunner/Mazel.

Whitaker, D. S., & Lieberman, M. A. (1964). *Psychotherapy through the group process*. Chicago: Aldine.

Williams, J. B. W., & Spitzer, R. L. (Eds.). (1984). *Psychotherapy research: Where are we and where should we go?* New York: Guilford Press.

Winston, A., Pinsker, H., & McCullough, L. (1986). A review of supportive psychotherapy. *Hospital and Community Psychiatry, 37*, 1105–1114.

Wolfenstein, M. (1966). How is mourning possible? *Psychoanalytic Study of the Child, 21*, 93–123.

Woods, M., & Melnick, J. (1979). A review of group therapy selection criteria. *Small Group Behavior, 10*, 155–175.

Worden, J. W. (1982). *Grief counseling and grief therapy: A handbook for the mental health practitioner*. New York: Springer.

Yalom, I. D. (1985). *The theory and practice of group psychotherapy* (3rd ed.). New York: Basic Books.

Yalom, I. D., & Vinogradov, S. (1988). Bereavement groups: Techniques and themes. *International Journal of Group Psychotherapy, 38*, 419–446.

Zisook, S. (Ed.). (1987). *Biopsychosocial aspects of bereavement*. Washington, DC: American Psychiatric Press.

Zisook, S., DeVaul, R. A., & Click, M. A. (1982). Measuring symptoms of grief and bereavement. *American Journal of Psychiatry, 139*, 1593–1594.

Zitrin, C. M., Klein, D. F., & Woerner, M. B. (1978). Behavior therapy, supportive psychotherapy, imipramine, and phobias. *Archives of General Psychiatry, 35*, 307–316.

Author Index

Subject Index